The KISSS Plan

4 Steps To Prevent or Reverse Type 2 Diabetes

Neil D'Silva

The KISSS Plan

First published in 2023
Bridge View Publishing
info@bridgeviewpublishing.com
www.bridgeviewpublishing.com
Paperback ISBN 979-8-40941-123-7
Hardcover ISBN 979-8-86494-378-6

The information in this book is provided for information and general purposes only, and is not intended to be nor should be construed as medical, health or clinical advice. While the author and the publisher has used their best efforts in preparing this book, they make no representations or warranties regarding the accuracy or completeness of the contents of this book and specifically disclaim any implied warranties of merchantability or fitness for a particular purpose.

Please contact a suitably qualified medical, dietary or other healthcare professional if you have an underlying health issue or have questions about the advice or strategies provided in this book. Neither the publisher nor the author shall be liable for any loss or damages, including but not limited to special, incidental, consequential, personal, or other damages.

A CIP catalogue record for this book is available from the British Library.

Without the written permission of the copyright holder, it is prohibited to reproduce any part of this book in material (including photocopying or storing in any medium by electronic means and whether transiently or incidentally to some other use of this publication), except under the Copyright, Design and Patents Act 1988.

The views and opinions expressed in this book are those of the author.

Copyright © 2024 by Neil D'Silva
www.diabetessolutions.co.uk
All rights reserved.
First Edition, November 2023
This Edition, March 2024

I dedicate this book to my family whom I love very much - to my wife Tracy, who has stood by me and never doubted that one day I would change the world; to my children Lauren, Alexander, James, and Melissa, who were my driving force for wanting to change and improve my life, and to my parents for making me the person I am today.

I would also like to thank Andrew Priestley for never giving up on the hope that, one day, I would write a book and share my knowledge with the world. I am not sure this book would have happened without his persistence and unwavering belief in me.

And to you, dear reader. Thank you for taking the time to read my book. I sincerely hope it changes your life.

Foreword

"I coach a lot of executives worldwide who are professionally qualified, ambitious and intelligent. They have big aspirations, and they do very demanding jobs. Although they are so successful in their business, when they step away from it, what I see (as almost the norm) is that they are overweight, they are out of shape, they are unfit, and their form of rest and relaxation might be a few beers in the evening, sitting in front of the television. They are inactive, they are not really moving, they are not doing anything that provides rest, recovery or restoration in any way, shape, or form - and figuratively speaking, they are knocking on an empty tank.

Now, this is okay, because you can go to a personal trainer or a nutritionist, and you can redesign the fuel that you are eating and your exercises and work it out that way. But some of my clients have exercise programmes and they have a perfect diet, and yet they are still overweight - they can't lose that weight and they really run low on energy. When you look at them, they look tired and exhausted.

I have been talking to Neil over a long period about the work he does with people who not only have what I described, but also present as potential candidates for type 2 diabetes. And then, when they have blood sugar checks done, type 2 diabetes is the issue.

I would say the biggest problem that I see is that they don't really understand what type 2 diabetes is, and they think "well okay, I've got type 2 diabetes and there is nothing more I can do about it". What I see is that Neil can take someone who has had that diagnosis and firstly help them manage it a lot more efficiently but, better than that, he's able to help his clients understand what type 2 diabetes is and how to reverse it.

This book is written for people who are at risk of developing type 2 diabetes or who have had a confirmed diagnosis - and they want a better understanding of what type 2 diabetes is and how they can manage it - but more importantly, how they could reverse that diagnosis.

I think this is an exciting book that Neil has put together. It is well researched; it is well written, there are years of study gone into it and years of working one-on-one with clients to do exactly what I've just described.

This is a book you should read slowly and make a lot of notes. You should most definitely follow the recommendations that Neil is suggesting from the very outset and take it seriously. If you have type 2 diabetes, there is every likelihood that you can get that condition under control if not reverse it - and that makes this a very important read."

Andrew Priestley

Contents

My Story 17
My 100 Million Mission 25
What Does "KISSS" Mean? 29
   Smart 31
   Simple 33
   Sustainable 37
The Four Cornerstones 39
How To Use This Book 43
Bonus Content 47
Setting SMART Goals 51
Understanding Your 'Why' 57
Unveiling Type 2 Diabetes 63
   What It Is and What It Is Not 65
   Some Startling Statistics 69
   The Implications 73
   Busting Some Type 2 Diabetes Myths 77
   Ignorance Is Not Bliss 83
   Spotting The Symptoms 85
Step 1: Nutrition 93
   Introduction 95
   The Journey of Glucose: From Plate to Cell 97
   Insulin and Blood Sugar Control 101
   The Sugar Addiction Cycle 103
   The Balancing Act 109

The Macronutrients	111
Carb Counting	139
Glycaemic Index and Glycaemic Load	143
Fibre	149
Omega 3 and Omega 6	153
Fruit	157
Fructose	161
Cakes, Biscuits, Drinks and Sweets	165
Healthy Snacking	169
Processed and Ultra Processed Foods	173
Whole Foods	177
Whole Grains	181
Hydration	185
Alcohol	191
Artificial Sweeteners	195
Sodium	201
Portion Sizes	205
Calories and Weight Management	209
Intermittent Fasting	215
The Dawn Phenomenon	221
The Somogyi Effect	225
Understanding Food Labels	231
The Traffic Light Food Label System	275
Type 2 Diabetes-Supporting Supplements	281
My Two Golden Rules	295
Step 1 Summary	299

- Step 2: Get Moving! 301
  - Introduction 303
  - Activity Boosts Energy Levels 305
  - Activity Supports Mental Health 309
  - Incorporating Exercise Into Daily Activity 311
  - Walking 317
  - Strength Training 321
  - Cardiovascular Exercise 325
  - Household Tasks: Movement in Disguise 329
  - Step 2 Summary 333
- Step 3: Holistic Wellbeing 335
  - Introduction 337
  - The Mind-Body Connection 339
  - Empowering the Mind for Physical Healing 345
  - Mindful Eating 349
  - The Importance Of Sleep 353
  - Stress Relieving Techniques 363
  - Journaling 365
  - Deep Breathing 369
  - Mindfulness 373
  - Step 3 Summary 377
- Step 4: Developing Sustainable Habits 379
  - Introduction 381
  - How We Form Habits 383
  - Establishing Positive Habits 387
  - Prioritising Consistency 393
  - Habit Linking 397
  - Celebrating Small Wins 401

Re-evaluating Traditional Rewards 405
Staying Adaptable 411
Anticipating Disruptions 415
Resetting Quickly 419
The Power of Positive Reinforcement 423
Bringing The 4 Steps Together 427
Bonus Pack 431
Free 15 Minute Zoom Consultation 433
Regular 121 Help 435
Free Online Reversal Assessment 437
Keep In Touch! 439
Closing Thoughts 441
Glossary 443
About The Author 463

Thank You

I would like to thank you for buying my book. My completing the book and sharing it with you and the rest of the world has been a labour of love for me - a project that has spanned over three years.

I am driven by a strong desire to use my personal and professional experiences with type 2 diabetes to help others facing similar struggles.

I struggled at times to find the motivation to continue writing this book and at those moments I reminded myself that helping others is a responsibility that I have embraced - and it would be remiss of me to not share with you the knowledge that has helped me to improve my health.

Even if you are the only one who benefits from my book, it will have been worth the time and effort.

I need to be really clear with you right from the outset and let you know that this is not a weight loss or 'fad' Diet (with a capital 'D') book. Not in any way, shape or form. I do not believe in 'Dieting' for many reasons – not least of which is that it is almost always unsustainable in the long term.

What this book is, however, is a comprehensive (but simple to understand) guide to help you get control of your blood sugars – and it therefore (depending on where you are with your health at this point) gives you the hope of reversing type 2 diabetes or indeed helping to reduce the risk of it happening.

I have observed over the years with my type 2 diabetic clients that making efforts to control their blood sugars and bringing them back into the 'normal' range often leads to a pleasant and welcome side effect of weight loss.

By focusing on blood sugar control, you are more likely to take sensible and sustainable actions to improve your health. People that focus solely on losing weight often do things that could never be condoned from a health improvement point of view - and I encourage you to focus first on improving your health, to trust the process and let any weight loss take care of itself.

Many books on type 2 diabetes focus primarily on diet - and there is a lot of truth in the saying that "you cannot out-exercise a bad diet". Indeed, as a nutritionist, much of my book is focused on nutrition, as you would expect. Preventing and reversing type 2 diabetes involves more than just food and drink, and this book covers those additional aspects.

If you are overweight, at risk of type 2 diabetes, are pre-diabetic or are a diagnosed type 2 diabetic – then this book is for you.

By taking the time to read my book, you are embarking on a journey towards better health.

First Things First…

The content of this book is for information only. It includes insights drawn from my knowledge and experiences gathered over the years and often reflects my views and opinions. I would like to clarify that I am not offering medical advice of any sort.

My simple goal is to improve your knowledge, to guide you in ways of reducing the risk of developing type 2 diabetes, or to reverse pre-diabetes / type 2 diabetes if you already have it, and inspire you to make positive changes in your life.

Before changing your diet, lifestyle, or current treatment plan it is essential that you consult with an appropriate healthcare professional first (for example, a nutritionist or your doctor).

I encourage you to conduct further research where you feel it would be helpful. This book was not intended to be a detailed analysis of specific topics. Its purpose is to provide enough basic understanding of the points covered so you can make changes.

Beyond that, I hope my book motivates you on the path of learning, to improving your health over the coming years and that you help and inspire your family, friends, and other people around you.

My Story

It is accepted that guidance from someone who has lived through a personal experience is more authentic and useful than advice from someone who has simply read a book on the topic - and I cannot think of anything truer when I look at my journey with my health and specifically with type 2 diabetes.

My name is Neil. Today, as a nutritionist and type 2 diabetes prevention/reversal specialist, my purpose in life is to help others by passing on the knowledge and tools to help them to either reduce the risk of developing type 2 diabetes, or to help them reverse the condition if they already have it.

You will note that I mention the words 'prevention' and 'reversal' – and not 'management'.

In my opinion, it is a 'management' mindset that keeps people stuck where they are – on escalating levels of medication, resigned to their fate and with a dwindling positivity for the future.

For those of you reading this book who do have type 2 diabetes - whilst full reversal is absolutely possible for you, you must accept that reversal is not guaranteed. However, I encourage you to develop a 'reversal' mindset as it leads to far more positive actions and to better results.

Even if you cannot reverse your type 2 diabetes, you will almost certainly benefit from improved overall health now and in the future.

Back in 2012...

When I think back to my journey, things were very different back in 2012 compared to now.

Back 2012, my life took an unexpected twist when my dad died at 66 of a complication related to type 2 diabetes. However, he was one of the tens of millions (likely hundreds of millions) of people around the world with undiagnosed type 2 diabetes - that is, he was living with the disease but was completely unaware of its existence or of the damage it was doing. This is a global issue and one that we will look at in more detail in step 1 of my plan.

Weeks after my dad's death and shortly after his funeral, I thought I would have a well-overdue health check done. Being conscious that, at 40, I wasn't getting any younger and, whilst I did not feel unhealthy, I felt that my health had perhaps declined over the preceding years.

I had a full health check. The results came back. It was not good news.

My blood sugar levels were significantly higher than normal. I also had high blood pressure together with raised cholesterol levels and a weight that pushed me into the realm of clinical obesity.

Not good. Not good at all.

I knew I was carrying too much weight. I also knew my diet was not great, and that I had led a pretty sedentary lifestyle. However, I had convinced myself – as many people do - that I was healthier than I really was and that whilst I wasn't 'good' with my diet and lifestyle habits, I did not think I was that bad either. Surely, like the proverbial ostrich with its head in the sand, I could continue avoiding the spectre of health problems if I simply convinced myself that these were things that happened to other people, and not to me.

Oh yes, and I reasoned that I 'was getting older' too, to excuse myself from taking any form of responsibility for my actions (or lack of, sometimes) because in my mind, getting older meant getting sicker and fatter.

Does that sound familiar?

Reality struck. I had a choice to take either a progressively increasing number of pills to keep me going or change my life.

Many people choose the former, and I respect that as their choice. However, I chose the latter. I am not anti-medication in any way - there are many occasions where medication is necessary and potentially lifesaving, but to me that was little more than 'painting my leaves green' - an illustration I would like to share with you for a moment, if I may:

Imagine for a moment - you have a tree in your garden and the leaves are turning brown. Clearly, the tree has a problem and is unwell. You call a tree specialist, and he turns up in his van, looks at the tree and says, "I know what is wrong and I can sort the problem out". Great, you think. He then pops back to his van and reappears with a can of green paint and a paintbrush and then paints the leaves of the tree green again. You would likely think that such actions would be baffling, that painting the leaves green again does little more than dealing with the symptoms of the problem and not the root cause (no pun intended!).

So, I wanted to do more than paint my leaves green. I wanted to find ways to get to the source of my problems and to deal with them sustainably.

I had to accept where I was, in order to move away from where I did not want to be. I also looked ahead to where I might be, health-wise, in ten or fifteen years' time if I did not take action.

So began my journey of change.

Through knowledge (and, more importantly, the application of that knowledge), persistent effort and determination to not be on potentially ever-increasing levels of medication nor to die young like my dad, I brought my blood sugar levels back into the normal range. I also brought my cholesterol and blood pressure levels back down too and lost a few stones in weight as a bonus!

It was as if I had unlocked a secret, a formula, a combination of knowledge, habits, and discipline.

"But what good is a secret if it remains hidden", I thought to myself. "There are literally hundreds of millions of people either heading towards where I once was with their own health or who are struggling right now, and who might benefit from what I have learnt and experienced."

So, transitioning into the field of nutrition was not just a professional shift for me, but a personal one, too. From that shift was born my "100 Million Mission" (which I will explain in a moment).

I have now made it my life's work to give hope to, and help, those at risk of type 2 diabetes, those who are pre-diabetic and those are currently living with the disease.

Type 2 diabetes is an endemic problem that now afflicts a significant proportion of the world, and it is only getting worse. It is humbling to think that, just perhaps, I can play a small part in reversing that trend.

In this book, I aim to share my experiences, insights, and knowledge.

Let this book be your companion. Allow it to help you improve your diet, lifestyle, habits, and mindset. Embrace it and benefit from what I have learnt over the years. The challenges I have faced and the victories I have celebrated can guide you, too.

I sincerely hope that this book helps you to understand why you need to move away from wherever you are right now in relation to type 2 diabetes, and the clarity and knowledge to show you how.

From the outset, I encourage you to have an open mind and to accept that you will probably need to change the way you view food, exercise, your lifestyle choices and general habits. Understand that this journey begins not with what you put in your mouth, but with what is between your ears. Get your thinking in the right place, and the rest will naturally follow.

As I mentioned, this is not a 'Diet' book, nor does it offer quick fixes (there are no sustainable quick fixes!). You are about to embark on a marathon and not a sprint. The journey of a thousand miles begins with the first step and today might just be the first day of the rest of your life… if you want it to be.

From personal experience, I can tell you that the destination of improved health is absolutely worth the effort the journey takes to get there.

To your good future health and prosperity,

Neil

PS. "You don't know what you don't know". If I only knew years ago what I know now, I may have been able to help my dad and perhaps he would still be here with me today. I acknowledge and accept the fact that I did not know then what I know now, and that I cannot change the past. I understand, however, that I can use my experience and knowledge to change my future and to improve the futures of others.

I recognise that if things had not transpired as they did back in August 2012, my life would have not taken the direction it has and it is unlikely that I would have fostered an interest in health and nutrition, and this book (one that I hope positively affects and changes the lives of hundreds, thousands, maybe millions of people across the world) would never have been written. Truth be told, I might not actually be here at all, or perhaps here but depending on a handful of drugs each day to keep me alive. A sobering thought, indeed.

That you are holding this book in your hands adds weight to the thought that maybe things happen for a reason.

My 100 Million Mission

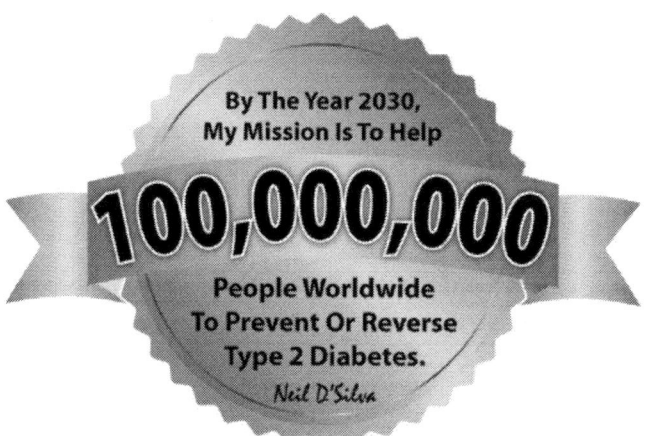

As you have learnt, my story in relation to type 2 diabetes includes moments of realisation that encouraged (arguably forced) me to take positive action. For me, one of those big moments was incredibly personal: the unexpected loss of my dad and then my health issues that came to light soon after. From acknowledging the thought that I cannot change the past, but I can influence the future, came my vision: my 100 Million Mission.

Every chapter you read, every piece of advice you take onboard and every positive change you implement from what you learn in this book is a step towards you improving your own health and wellbeing. If my book helps you, then please tell others about it.

Beyond that, I would like to see a world where no-one experiences the pain and loss I have gone through, and where we consign type 2 diabetes to the annuls of history.

By equipping yourself with the knowledge within this book (and putting that knowledge into practice where you feel you need to), you are not only helping to safeguard your own health, but can also influence those around you. You are helping to demonstrate that type 2 diabetes is not an inevitable destiny (as is, sadly, often accepted these days), but a preventable - and reversible - condition.

Remember, my 100 Million Mission is not just about numbers – it is about real people, real stories, real lives improved and real lives saved. Every single person I can help in relation to type 2 diabetes adds another chapter to my 100 Million Mission.

By spreading awareness about type 2 diabetes and sharing the knowledge from this book, you are helping fight against the disease.

Each person you touch with your story, every conversation you spark and each recommendation you make, inches us closer to the mission of improving countless millions of lives. Every journey, including mine, began with that first, single step.

Your commitment to reading this book, taking action where necessary and supporting its cause by sharing what you learn with others is an integral part of the realisation of my 100 Million Mission.

With every step you take towards healthier choices, you are contributing to a shared vision - a world where stories like mine (and my dad's) are a thing of the past.

I am striving for a collective movement towards better global wellbeing and type 2 diabetes awareness, not just your personal health.

This is the heart of my 100 Million Mission. It is now time to turn the pages and rewrite the future of global health.

Let's change the world together.

What Does "KISSS" Mean?

The subject of nutrition and health can often feel overwhelming at the best of times. With countless diets and health fads popping up every year, it is important to sift through the noise and the gimmicks, and to embrace what truly has stood the test of time.

Enter my 'KISSS' philosophy
KISSS is my acronym for 'Keep It Smart, Simple and Sustainable' and this philosophy has served me well. Irrespective of your age, cultural background, or dietary preferences, the principles of making smart, simple and sustainable choices can benefit you, too. You can adapt and mould the three S's - smart, simple, and sustainable choices - to fit your individual lifestyle, dietary habits, and health objectives.

Not that following my KISSS philosophy is necessarily easy. As the saying goes… "if it were easy, then everyone would do it".

Like me, you are a human being with imperfections, flawed thinking, ingrained habits, temptations, and lots of other baggage that make 'doing the right thing' challenging.

What I will stress is that to succeed in the KISSS philosophy, you must pursue progress and never perfection. Trust that this book will help you change your ingrained habits.

You will start to not only make better choices that will help you form new habits, but will understand the reasons why.

Remember, knowledge is not power. **Applied knowledge is power.**

With that in mind, let us set down some foundations and explore each of my three 'S' principles.

Smart

It is important to be 'smart' when it comes to decisions that relate to your health, and the 'smart' facet of my KISSS philosophy is all about making informed choices which are driven by knowledge.

Embarking on a journey to prevent or reverse type 2 diabetes without knowledge is like trying to navigate a ship without a compass. Understanding the basics is crucial, such as the role of insulin, how different foods affect blood sugar, the importance of regular monitoring and more. Knowledge will empower you to make informed decisions.

Personalisation over generalisation
Your journey - whether that is prevention or reversal of type 2 diabetes, is unique to you. Factors like age, genetics, lifestyle, and even sleep quality and stress levels play a role in how the disease progresses. Therefore, it is wise to personalise your strategies and see this book as your guide to help you make smarter decisions.

Prioritising holistic wellbeing
Remember to look at the bigger picture of your health, beyond just controlling blood sugar levels. This includes recognising how your physical, emotional and mental health interact with each other.

Leveraging technology

Today's technology can make monitoring type 2 diabetes straight forward. Smart use of technology might involve utilising an online food diary to track nutrition, setting reminders for medication or insulin doses, or using a Constant Glucose Monitor (CGM) to monitor blood sugar levels in real-time. These tools, when used effectively, can make management of blood sugars more efficient, and reversal possible.

Continuous learning and adaptation

The field of nutrition is ever developing and I encourage you to stay updated, be open to learning and be willing to adapt your strategies, considering new knowledge. I also welcome you to sign up to my regular free email updates at **www.diabetessolutions.co.uk/subscribe.**

Setting realistic goals

'Smart' is also about setting achievable targets. Whether that is related to weight loss, your blood sugar levels or dietary changes - having clear, realistic goals provides direction. Reaching these milestones also gives you a sense of achievement, which motivates you to continue.

Being 'smart' in the context of my KISSS philosophy is about combining knowledge with intuition, using evidence-based practices, personalising strategies, and leveraging the resources around you.

Simple

We live in an age of information overload, which creates a challenge in being able to cut through the noise - and when that relates to our health, that is not ideal.

I believe in simplicity. If a new routine or process is too difficult, it can lead to relapse and disappointment, bringing you back to square one. Keeping things simple and having a straightforward, uncomplicated approach is critical.

The 'simple' aspect of my KISSS philosophy promotes the idea that, in many cases, the most effective strategies are those that are easy to understand, implement and - more importantly - maintain.

Decluttering nutritional advice

Understanding nutrition, especially in relation to type 2 diabetes, can feel like navigating a maze. However, committing to simple changes day after day, week after week, often yields the most significant results.

Instead of fixating on every nutrient or new diet fad, I suggest you prioritise the basics of healthy eating. This includes eating whole foods, cutting back on processed foods, limiting refined sugar, and maintaining a balanced diet. These simple steps can improve your blood sugar control and overall health.

Regular, manageable exercise

The thought of a strenuous workout regime can be daunting for many people. But simplicity in exercise (and incorporating movement that can be implemented every day with little effort) is both achievable and beneficial for most people. The key is consistency over intensity.

Progress and not perfection!

Streamlined monitoring

Frequent health checks and blood sugar monitoring is important for those with type 2 diabetes. Setting regular schedules, using user-friendly monitoring devices and maintaining a straightforward log of results demystifies the process, makes it less tedious and in conjunction with a food diary, will give you a great understanding of how what you eat and drink affects your blood sugar levels.

Setting clear, achievable goals

Big goals can feel overwhelming, so break them down into smaller steps.

For example:
- Instead of aiming to lose a large amount of weight in a year, focus on losing a manageable amount each month.
- Instead of focusing on complete type 2 diabetes reversal, aim to reduce your average bloods sugars at your next HBA1C test by 10%.

- Of course, you will still want to stay focused on your ultimate goal(s), but they will not feel so out of reach as you make step-by-step progress.

Imagine being at the base camp of a mountain, with the goal of reaching the summit. Yes, it is great to look up at the summit and to where you want to be but, at the same time, that can feel very daunting and perhaps demoralising to be constantly reminded of where you currently are. It is good to keep in mind your ultimate goal, but to focus on the next step you need to take towards it, and then the step after that. By working on step-by-step progress, a bit like walking a mountain trail, you will be less likely to slip off.

Uncomplicated meal preparation
Meal planning does not have to involve intricate recipes with a host of ingredients. Often, the healthiest meals are simple, with minimal ingredients and easy preparation methods.

I have put together over 100 healthy breakfast, lunch and evening meal recipes, and you can download them for free at
www.diabetessolutions.co.uk/tkp-bonuspack

Sustainable

At the heart of preventing or reversing type 2 diabetes lies a profound truth – it is not just about making changes; it is about making those changes last.

The health and nutrition industry is flooded with so-called 'Diet' companies that promise to transform your body. Sadly, most of these 'magic-bullet' solutions disappoint and even fewer are sustainable in the long term. Perhaps you've tried these before and felt the hope, temporary progress, and subsequent disappointment as you returned to your starting point (or worse)?

I believe that the key to better health lies, not just in making changes, but ensuring those changes are sustainable - ideally for the rest of your life.

Understanding sustainability in health
At its essence, sustainability in health is about embedding practices you can maintain over your lifetime - a shift from the short-lived enthusiasm of unachievable new-year resolutions or fad-diets, to cultivating habits that weave seamlessly into the fabric of your daily routines. There is a temptation to lean towards promises of rapid results and, sadly, over the years, the so-called 'Diet' market has been more than happy to accommodate those looking for quick fixes.

While these fad-diets might offer passing benefits, they lack longevity. Quick fixes, either in the form of drastic diets or intensive workout programmes, may provide short-term outcomes, but by their nature they are often challenging to maintain - leading to cycles of relapse.

A sustainable approach recognises that as your life changes, so do your needs and routines. What might be sustainable at one life stage might need tweaking in another. Regularly revisiting and adjusting your health strategies ensures they remain relevant and effective.

Celebrating milestones

Recognising and celebrating progress (no matter how big or small) can significantly boost your motivation to stay on track. When you pause to acknowledge the positive shifts in your health, energy levels, or even mood, it fuels your commitment to continue.

The 'sustainable' component of my KISSS philosophy highlights the importance of long-term, enduring changes in preventing or reversing type 2 diabetes. Avoiding the pitfalls of quick fixes, embracing incremental changes, fostering emotional wellbeing, evolving with time, grounding in education and celebrating milestones are the key elements that define sustainability.

The Four Cornerstones

In a world saturated with fleeting health trends and overwhelming information, the pathway to understanding, preventing, or reversing type 2 diabetes can seem daunting. I have structured this book to change that - offering you a holistic, understandable, and actionable blueprint.

I could have made my book shorter, maybe cutting short the nutritional knowledge covered in step 1 or maybe focusing on just diet and nothing else - but I consciously chose not to. Step 1 just so happens to be the longest of the 4 steps - and with good reason. Not improving your understanding of nutrition and make better dietary choices is like neglecting to lay a solid foundation when building a house. You can build a house on land without putting down foundations, which is quicker and cheaper in the short term. But we know that strategy is neither smart nor sustainable.

Step 1. Nutritional knowledge and understanding
I strongly believe that understanding nutrition is the first step towards making a lasting change. Without first grasping the foundations of the 'what' and the 'why' of type 2 diabetes prevention and reversal, the 'how' becomes little more than an instruction manual.

The "do as you are instructed" model is the one that sets you up for long-term failure, but when you make choices based on knowledge, you will almost certainly make better decisions.

"Give a man a fish and feed him for a day. Teach him how to fish and feed him for life."

Step 1 guides you through first the nutritional what and the why, and shows you how.

Remember, knowledge, if left on the shelf, does nothing but gather dust.

Applied knowledge is power.

Step 2. Get moving!
By the end of step 1, you will have a good basic understanding of nutrition, and you will also have put together your own list of action points to help you apply that knowledge in your day-to-day life. As we know, when it comes to controlling blood sugar levels, making better informed dietary choices is one of the most powerful and life-changing tools available in your toolbox.

However, 'good health' is holistic - it is interconnected with your physical and your emotional health. So, in step 2 we are going to get you moving, and look at ways to increase activity to improve your physical health.

Step 3: Holistic wellbeing

Your wellbeing is a harmonious blend of the mental, emotional and physical, as we will find out in step 3. A fragmented approach is unlikely to give you lasting results and again, this is where I feel a lot of so-called 'Diet' plans fall short – they focus just on diet and little else.

I aim to redress that balance and to help you, as we look at the other areas of your life that all contribute towards the definition of "being healthy".

Step 4: Creating sustainable habits for life

Health is a lifelong journey, not a destination. While quick fixes might seem appealing, it is the sustainable habits that promise long-term health dividends. Sustainable habits ensure that the positive changes you make can be lifelong.

In step 4, we will look at how you can build habits. This step will help you put in to practise all that you have learnt in steps 1 to 3, and make them last a lifetime.

Perhaps easier said than done - but achievable, nonetheless.

What sets this book apart?

Most books on the market merely present fragmented solutions or are overly complicated. My intention when writing this book was to root it in the ethos of holistic health and to write it in a language that is easily understood - and, more importantly, easy to put into action.

It does not just tell; it shows. It does not just inform; it guides. It is a consolidated tool that, if followed, looks to change your life and lives around the world for the better.

Knowledge, as I have pointed out, is only valuable if acted upon. It is like a locked treasure chest. The application of the knowledge is the key. This book works hard to ensure that the treasure, once unlocked, is of benefit to you.

I encourage you to embrace The KISSS Plan with an open heart and a committed mindset.

At the end of the book, I have included a glossary of many type 2 diabetes and health related terms you may choose to refer to as you progress through. Please make good use of it. I appreciate readers will have differing levels of nutritional and diabetic knowledge and so I have tried to keep the book as simple to understand as possible.

How To Use This Book

When I came up with the concept of the KISSS Plan, I wanted to create a blueprint that anyone could follow regardless of where they might be in relation to type 2 diabetes. Whether you are at risk of developing type 2 diabetes, are pre-diabetic or are diagnosed with the disease - every section holds value.

I've organised the book into 4 steps that you can work through in order or jump to topics that catch your attention.

In step 1, we begin with the foundation of good health - nutrition. After that, step 2 covers movement and exercise, with step 3 looking deeper at the holistic areas that contribute to good health. Finally, step 4 examines how we can bring it all together to can create new, better and sustainable habits that will last you a lifetime.

Taking notes, and the "Priority 1" and "Priority 2" Action Points
It is unlikely that I know you personally and even less likely that I know your personal situation, your habits, your lifestyle, your unique relationship with type 2 diabetes or the exact reason you have chosen to read my book. I aim to cover all the major relevant topics related to type 2 diabetes prevention/reversal and blood sugar control, to cover all the bases. Some of these topics may not apply to you, but the chances are that many will. Pay specific attention to the subjects that are relevant,

and please do still read through the less relevant areas to gain a more complete overview.

As you progress through the book, there are several 'Action Points' at the end of most sections, and these are classified as "Priority 1" and "Priority 2":

>> ACTION POINTS - PRIORITY 1 <<

*Not all 'Priority 1' action points will apply to you, but most likely, many will be. If they are, consider them non-negotiable and the most important. On the 'Action Points' worksheet (in the **free downloadable bonus pack** that I have created for you), you will notice that there is a column marked 'Priority'. As you list each 'must-do' action point that you will work on, prioritise them either as a '1' (being the most important to you) or a '2'. Once you have completed all of your 'Priority 1' action points, you can then work on those that are 'Priority 2'.*

www.diabetessolutions.co.uk/tkp-bonuspack

>> ACTION POINTS - PRIORITY 2 <<

As the title suggests, in addition to the 'Priority 1' action points, the 'Priority 2' action points are also good to work on where relevant - although they should ideally not take priority.

Please revisit relevant sections as your journey progresses and the weeks and months pass by, and pick out new and additional action points to work on. This should be a very fluid process and I encourage you to personalise how you make best use of the content in the book to fit your needs, lifestyle, and other commitments. There is no 'one size fits all', however, the more 'Action Points' you put in to practise, the more likely you are to experience noticeable results. They are what will take you from where you are right now to where you want to be. After all, isn't that the reason you picked up this book in the first place?

Before we dive in to step 1, I would like to offer you some free bonus content that will help you as you progress through the book. After that, we will look at how you can set SMART goals, and also how you can really dig deep and establish some strong 'whys' - the reasons for wanting to improve your health.

Bonus Content

To help you get the most from my book, please download the free bonus pack.

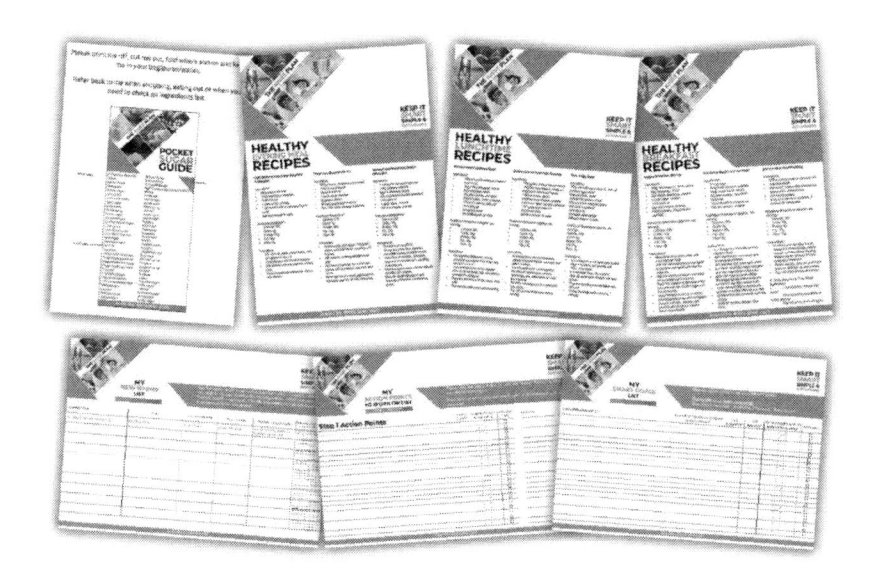

Over 100 free healthy breakfast, lunch and evening meal recipes

As you will learn in step 1, one cornerstone of preventing and reversing type 2 diabetes is nutrition. To make this process more enjoyable, I have prepared a collection of over 100 delicious and healthy breakfast, lunch and evening meal recipes. These recipes are specifically crafted to support balanced blood sugar levels and overall wellbeing.

Free SMART goals worksheet

SMART goals will form a vital part of your journey to better health. To make this process easier for you, I have created a 'SMART goals' template for you to note down your own personal goals. Whether you are focusing on blood sugar control, weight loss, dietary changes or increasing physical activity, this template will guide you in turning your aspirations into actionable and attainable goals.

Free sugar names pocket guide

Navigating food labels can be a challenge, especially when it comes to identifying hidden sugars. This handy pocket-sized guide provides you with a list of alternative names for sugar commonly found on ingredient lists. From sucrose to high fructose corn syrup to molasses and more, you will spot added sugars more easily with this guide, helping you make healthier choices while shopping.

Free 'Action Points' worksheet

Taking action is the key to success. You will no doubt learn a lot as you progress through the book, but knowledge is not power - the true power comes from applying that knowledge. The 'Action Points' worksheet helps you translate the knowledge you gain as you journey through the book into actionable steps. By recording your progress and staying accountable, you will be well on your way to achieving your health goals.

Free 'Change Your Habits' worksheet

In step 4, we cover habits, loops and linking. The free 'Change Your Habits' worksheet is an invaluable tool for this section, and can help you identify and then change habits that are not working against your health interests.

How to access your bonus pack

To access your bonus content, simply visit the following link:

www.diabetessolutions.co.uk/tkp-bonuspack

Once there, you will find the download link for the pack. Pop your name and email address in the form, and I will email the PDF's to you. Please save them to your computer and print them out, as needed.

I encourage you to make the most of these resources, as they complement the contents of the book, and help you get the most from it as you read through.

Setting SMART Goals

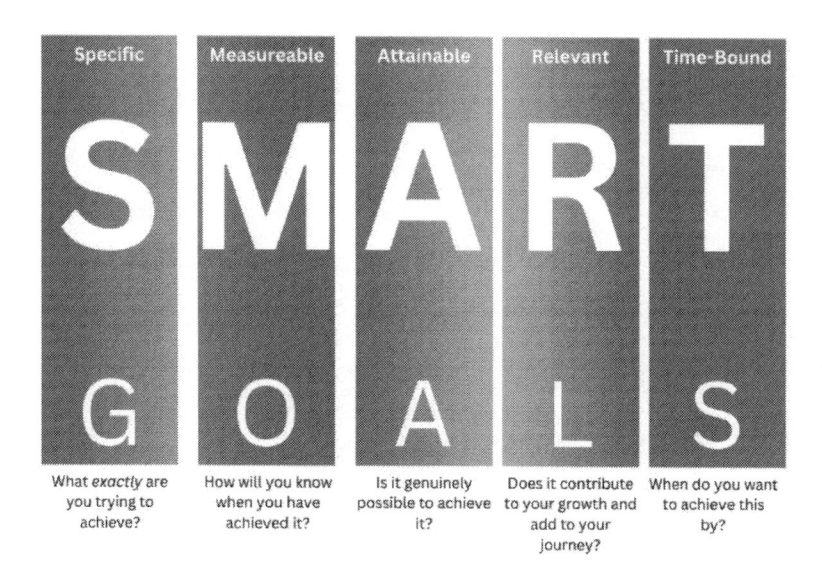

Specific	Measureable	Attainable	Relevant	Time-Bound
What *exactly* are you trying to achieve?	How will you know when you have achieved it?	Is it genuinely possible to achieve it?	Does it contribute to your growth and add to your journey?	When do you want to achieve this by?

Beginning your journey to better health and blood sugar control is like embarking on a quest. Like adventurers who plan their path and destination, having a clear plan will be beneficial for you as well.

Your own health map must be designed with SMART goals in mind.

SMART = Specific, Measurable, Attainable, Relevant, Time-bound.

SMART provides structure and direction for making goals achievable and sustainable.

You may have heard of SMART goals before, and indeed may well have used them to set and reach goals in the past. Alternatively, this may be the first time you have come across the concept.

The benefits of SMART goals

One of the primary benefits of SMART goals is their ability to bring clarity and focus. They help you define **'S'pecifically** what you want to achieve and when, and act as your compass - ensuring that you stay on course. When your path is clearly laid out in front of you, you are more likely to stay committed and motivated.

SMART goals are **'M'easurable**, which means you can gauge your progress as you go along. This is important, as it provides you with a sense of accomplishment and helps you understand what is working and what requires change. For example, if your goal is to lower your HBA1C level, you can regularly measure your progress through blood tests, enabling you to track your journey towards better blood sugar control.

'A'ttainable goals are important for helping you to maintain motivation. Unrealistic goals can lead to frustration and a sense of failure. So, strike a balance between challenging and attainable objectives, and allow yourself to progress without becoming disheartened by unreachable targets.

SMART goals keep you rooted in to your health objectives and they ensure your efforts are **'R'elevant** to your values, your priorities, and your long-term vision. This relevance is essential because it helps you see 'why' your goals matter in the grand scheme of your health and wellbeing.

'T'ime-bound' helps you to stay focused and guards against procrastination. Setting a clear deadline for when you want to achieve your goal makes it more tangible and actionable.

How to set SMART goals

Specific: Start by making your goal as specific as possible. Ask yourself what, why, and how. Instead of a vague goal like "I want to eat healthier," make it specific by saying "I will eat five servings of fruits and vegetables every day to improve my nutrition." This specificity paints a clear picture of what you are striving to accomplish.

Measurable: Ensure your goals can be quantified. This allows you to track your progress. For instance, if your goal relates to physical activity, specify how many minutes you will exercise each day or week. If your goal is related to diet, define the maximum number of grams of added sugar you will limit yourself to each day.

Attainable: To ensure that your goals are realistic and attainable, consider your circumstances, resources and limitations. For example, setting a goal to lose 10kg in a month may not be attainable nor healthy, so instead aim for gradual and sustainable changes that are realistic.

Relevant: Align your goal with your long-term objectives. If your primary goal is to reverse type 2 diabetes, for example, focus on setting sub-goals related to blood sugar control, your diet, and exercise.

Time-Bound: Set a specific timeframe for your goal. This could be a daily, weekly, or monthly deadline. For example, "I will reduce the number of teaspoons of sugar in my coffee/tea from two to zero within 4 weeks." This time-bound element adds a sense of urgency and prevents you from indefinitely postponing your efforts.

Please download, print off and make good use of my free SMART goals template that I have prepared for you at
www.diabetessolutions.co.uk/tkp-bonuspack

>> ACTION POINTS - PRIORITY 1 <<

Reflect on your health and identify specific areas where you would like to make improvements

Find a quiet, comfortable space and consider different aspects of your health like diet, exercise, blood sugar management, and well-being. Set at least one SMART goal in each area. Ask yourself questions like, "what areas do I want to improve?" or "where might I face challenges in my health journey?" Make a written note of these. Reflecting on this will help you identify specific areas for positive changes and personalised SMART goals.

Using the downloadable template, create SMART goals for the areas you have noted above - ensuring they are Specific, Measurable, Achievable, Relevant, and Time-bound
Setting SMART goals is a practical process, so begin by choosing the areas you want to improve in. Then, make your goals…
Specific *(by clearly defining what you want to achieve),*
Measurable *(by including details like quantities, duration, or specific metrics to track your progress),*
Achievable *(by considering your current capabilities, limitations and resources),*
Relevant *(to your overall health journey), and finally*
Time-bound *(deadlines create a sense of urgency and commitment).*

For example, if your goal is to improve your physical activity, then specify "I will walk for 30 minutes every day, starting from tomorrow." This approach will help you craft effective, actionable goals aligned with your 'why.'

Break down your larger goals into smaller, manageable steps

To achieve your SMART goals, it is essential to break them down into smaller, manageable steps. This approach makes your goals less overwhelming and more attainable. For instance, if your goal is weight loss, break it down into monthly weight loss targets. By focusing on achievable milestones, you can celebrate your progress along the way, which boosts your motivation and reinforces your commitment to your 'why'.

Regularly track your progress and celebrate your achievements along the way

Tracking your progress is an important aspect of achieving your SMART goals, so start by keeping a journal or a digital document where you can record your achievements - being sure to acknowledge even the smallest successes (such as sticking to your daily exercise routine or making healthier food choices). This practice not only keeps you motivated, but also reinforces your commitment to your goals. By consistently tracking and celebrating your accomplishments along the way, you will maintain a positive mindset and stay on course to achieving your long-term objectives. Remember, every step in the right direction is a step in the right direction!

Be flexible, and willing to adjust your goals as needed

Your health needs and priorities may change over time, so periodically review your goals and assess whether they still align with your current situation and objectives, and make modifications that better suit your changing circumstances.

Understanding Your 'Why'

Understanding your 'why' is like having a sturdy rudder on the ship of your life - it is the guiding force that can propel you forward. With a strong 'why' you are more likely to find success on this journey and reach your ultimate goal.

At its core, your 'why' is the essence of your purpose - the fundamental reason (or reasons) driving your desire for change. It goes straight to the heart of what truly matters to you.

To illustrate this, allow me to introduce you to Sarah. Sarah is a woman in her mid-50s and is pre-diabetic. Her doctor has advised her to make dietary and lifestyle changes to reverse her pre-diabetes. At first, she enthusiastically embraces her journey of healthier eating and regular exercise. Her dietary and lifestyle changes last for a couple of weeks, but then she loses interest as her efforts are based on nothing more than being told what to do by her doctor. The underlying problem is that Sarah has not taken the time to establish her own clear reason 'why' she needs to make changes - and her efforts quickly lose momentum.

Sarah then takes some time to reflect on her 'why' and she sets herself some SMART goals. She realises that her desire for better health is not just about lowering her blood sugar or losing a few pounds. Her 'why' is deeply rooted in her longing to be actively involved in her grandchildren's lives for as long as possible, to witness them growing up, to share in their joys and milestones and who knows - maybe even get to meet her great-grandchildren someday. This revelation transforms Sarah's motivation and gives her a profound sense of purpose. Suddenly, making healthier choices becomes not just a task, but a passionate pursuit. Her 'why' ignites her determination and fuels her journey to better health.

The psychology of 'why'

We humans are purpose-driven beings. We thrive when we have a sense of direction and meaning in our lives. Understanding your own 'why' taps into that psychology of motivation, and can provide you with focus, it can align your actions with your values, it can help you be resilient, it can make your goals more meaningful, and it shifts your focus from short-term gains to long-term benefits.

Unearthing your 'why'

Discovering your 'why' is a deeply introspective and personal process, but it is vital.

Begin by reflecting on your core values - what principles and beliefs are most important to you in life? These values often hold the key to your 'why.'

Then consider your aspirations and goals. What health goals do you want to achieve? Be as specific as possible. For example, if reversing type 2 diabetes is your goal, ask yourself why it is important to you.

That could be not wanting to deal with additional complications as the disease advances, it might be wanting to see your children grow up, it could be that you want to enjoy a healthy and active old age. Your aspirations are personal to you, and they should motivate you to want to make the necessary changes.

Next, pay attention to your emotions. When you think about your health journey, what emotions arise? Is there a sense of urgency, a longing for something better, or a desire for liberation from health-related constraints?

And finally, close your eyes and visualise your life with improved health. What does it feel to be free of type 2 diabetes? How will it feel when you no longer have to take medication? How worthwhile will the effort have been when you see your grandchildren being born and you get to watch them grow up? Picture the positive changes in your daily life, relationships, and overall wellbeing. This visualisation can help solidify your 'why.'

>> ACTION POINTS - PRIORITY 1 <<

Journal your 'Why': Dedicate a journal or digital document to explore your 'Why'
Begin by finding a journal or note-taking app dedicated to your health journey. Start with a clear title like "My Reason Why." Next, take a moment to reflect on your core values, aspirations, and emotions

related to your health goals and write these down. Be honest and specific about what truly matters to you. For example, if one of your values is "family," you might write about your desire to be actively present in your family's life as a motivation for better health. As you progress on your health journey, regularly revisit your journal to track your evolving 'why' and stay connected to your purpose. This simple practice can provide profound clarity and motivation.

Set clear goals: Transform your 'why' into SMART goals

Turning your 'why' into actionable goals is a powerful way to make change. Start by identifying your broader health goals, such as improving blood sugar control or losing weight. Then, break these down into Specific, Measurable, Attainable, Relevant, and Time-bound. For example, instead of a vague goal like "I want to lose weight," make it specific by saying, "I aim to lose 5kg in the next three months." Next, create a list of smaller, manageable steps that will lead you to those SMART goals. These could include changes in your daily routine, like adding a 20-minute walk after dinner or substituting sugary snacks with healthier options. By breaking your 'why' into clear and achievable steps, you will develop a clear roadmap to follow, making your goals more attainable and less overwhelming.

>> ACTION POINTS - PRIORITY 2 <<

Celebrate milestones: As you progress toward your goals, celebrate your achievements

When you achieve a goal or reach a milestone, take a moment to acknowledge your accomplishments. Recognising and celebrating your achievements, no matter how small, builds confidence and reinforces your progress towards your long-term goals. This is the positive reinforcement that will keep you motivated.

Create a vision board: A visual representation of your 'why' can be powerful

Creating a vision board to visualise your 'why' is a creative and effective tool. Start by gathering magazines, images, and words that resonate with your health goals and your 'why'. Look for visuals in magazines or print off images from relevant internet searches that inspire you and that connect with your values and aspirations. Get a poster board or a large piece of paper, glue, scissors, and markers. Begin to arrange and glue the images onto the board and arrange them in a way that feels meaningful to you. Once your vision board is complete, place it somewhere visible where you will see it daily. This visual representation will serve as a constant reminder of your 'why,' and will help you stay motivated and act in alignment with your goals.

Unveiling Type 2 Diabetes

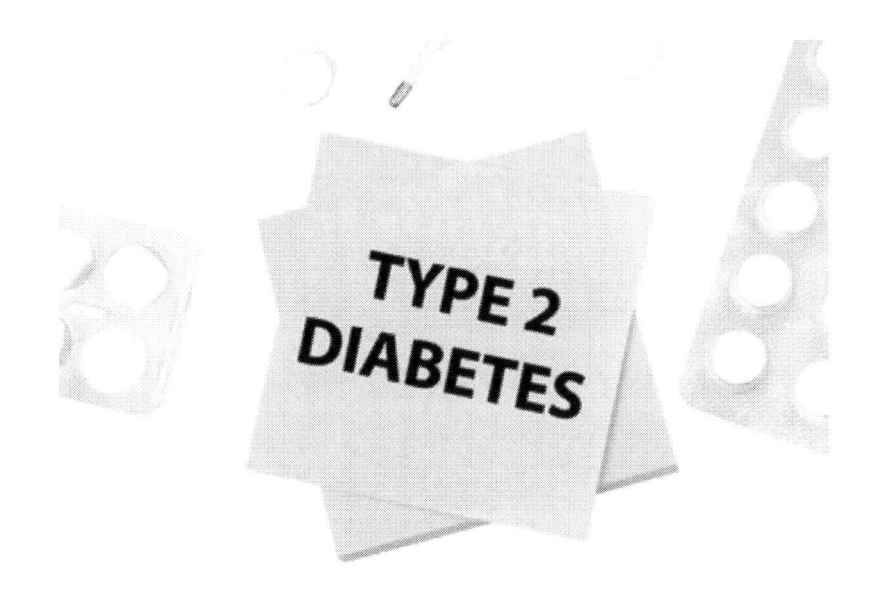

What It Is and What It Is Not

'Type 2 diabetes' is an often misunderstood. Lots of people have heard of 'diabetes' from the media and others around them, but are rarely aware even that there are many types, let alone what 'type 2' is.

This concerns me, as to stand a chance of prevention or reversal, we really need to understand what type 2 diabetes is. At this point then, before I look to improve your knowledge and establish practical ways for you to put the KISSS Plan into action, it would be good to take a closer look at what type 2 diabetes is, unearth some facts and dispel some myths.

The core concept
At the centre of the type 2 diabetes epidemic is glucose, and chances are you have probably heard of it. Glucose is a simple sugar derived from the food (specifically carbohydrates) that you eat. Glucose is not the villain of the piece in and of itself, as your body uses glucose a primary source of energy.

For glucose to be utilised by the body effectively, it needs to be transported from the bloodstream into your body's cells. This is where insulin, a hormone produced by the pancreas, comes into play.

In type 2 diabetes, there are problems with this normally straightforward process. Either the pancreas is not producing enough insulin or, more commonly, the cells become 'resistant' to insulin's effects (imagine insulin being the key to the locked door on our cells, and the key no longer fits properly or the lock is blocked).

This inability to put the glucose where it needs to be leads to elevated blood glucose levels (hyperglycaemia) which, when left unchecked, can cause widespread damage to pretty much every system of the body.

(Do not worry about trying to take all of this on board at this stage. I am going to walk you through these topics in Step 1).

What type 2 diabetes is not: temporary high blood sugar

It is important to understand the difference between occasional spikes in blood sugar levels and chronic hyperglycaemia. While it is natural for blood sugar levels to rise after we eat (and specifically when we eat carbohydrate-rich meals), in healthy individuals this is brought back down to normal levels within an hour or two by the function of insulin, as noted.

The definition of type 2 diabetes is the long-term inability for the body to manage these raised blood sugar levels effectively.

The underlying causes

There is not one single contributing cause that has been isolated as the development of type 2 diabetes, although your diet is one of, if not the biggest, factor ("you are what you eat").

Let us briefly look at some of the other influential factors aside from our diet:

Lifestyle

Sedentary lifestyles and carrying too much weight (particularly around the belly) are significant risk factors. Excessive body fat (particularly 'visceral' fat that can accumulate around the organs) produces chemicals that can interfere with insulin production, and its effectiveness.

Age

The risk increases with age, particularly after 45, although it is now becoming more common in younger populations because of lifestyle shifts. Once known as "the middle-aged person's disease", type 2 diabetes is now becoming more common in children, some of whom are tragically of pre-school age. In fact, it was once pretty much unheard of for children to be diagnosed with type 2 diabetes, further emphasising the need for education and action.

Ethnicity

Some groups, like South Asian, African-Caribbean and Middle Eastern individuals, are at a higher risk of developing type 2 diabetes.

Genetics

Having a family history of type 2 diabetes can increase the risk, but diet and lifestyle play a far bigger role than genetics. I take this as being a positive, as once a person learns type 2 diabetes is not necessarily genetic, then that can inspire them to take action to reverse it.

Some Startling Statistics

Type 2 diabetes has now become a global (and arguably out of control) epidemic. The impact it is having across the world underscores the urgent need for better awareness, intervention, and a collective approach towards prevention and reversal.

I do not want to spend too much time on the stats, as that is not the purpose of this book (and besides, the numbers are constantly changing anyway). However, it is useful to have an overview of the scale of the problem - so let us have a look at some background information.

The global surge
Type 2 diabetes has seen explosive growth in recent decades, with close to 500 million people now diagnosed with the disease at the time of writing. To put this in perspective, despite worldwide governmental intervention, that is nearly five times the amount compared to 1980. Clearly, we have a problem, and one that seems to be only getting worse.

What is equally alarming is that this increase is not confined to so-called affluent nations. We now witness emerging economies and developing countries facing a steep rise in type 2 diabetes cases, caused predominantly because of shifts in lifestyles, rapid urbanisation and changes in dietary patterns (linked, in part at least, to the adoption of the unhealthy 'western' diet with its high fat, high sugar, high salt, fast food culture).

The silent majority - undiagnosed cases

While the official figures are frightening for most people, they are likely just the tip of the very unpleasant iceberg. Right now, many people are living with undiagnosed type 2 diabetes, completely unaware of the challenges that lie ahead. It is thought that **almost half** of the people with type 2 diabetes across the world are **yet to be diagnosed.**

*That takes us to well over **one billion people.***

Tangible complications

Type 2 diabetes is not a standalone condition – and by that, I mean it is a precursor to a range of other potentially serious health issues including cardiovascular disease, stroke, kidney disease and eye problems that can lead to blindness. Then there is nerve damage that can ultimately lead to limb amputation. The domino effect of type 2 diabetes is **very** real and can be **very** life changing.

Mortality rates: a grim picture

Because of the complications associated with type 2 diabetes, it is now a leading cause of death (and premature death) worldwide. Every death is not just a sad statistic, but an avoidable sad statistic. It underscores the urgent need for improved knowledge and action. Despite efforts, health services and governments have not been able to stop the rise of type 2 diabetes. We need to take personal responsibility for our health.

The economic toll

Beyond health, type 2 diabetes puts a significant strain on economies across the world. The direct costs of treatment, medication and health services, coupled with the indirect costs like loss of productivity, absenteeism and premature mortality, have a tremendous impact. At the time of writing, it is estimated that the annual global health expenditure on type 2 diabetes and type 2 diabetes-related complications is near US$825 billion – a figure likely to increase to over US$1 trillion per year in the coming years.

What does the future hold?

Looking back over recent decades and observing the trend in recent years, the trajectory of type 2 diabetes cases is likely to continue to rise. It is estimated that by 2045, nearly 700 million people could be diagnosed with type 2 diabetes (and remember, that is only the people that have been actually diagnosed).

I remind you that whilst these are truly astounding numbers, every one of those is a human being - with real struggles, real challenges, real suffering and potentially a real premature death. The numbers alone scream out for better awareness, improved understanding and, most importantly, a total commitment to positive action.

The Implications

We now know that about 50% of those with type 2 diabetes have yet to be diagnosed, and this is a massive problem.

Left unchecked (or undiagnosed), type 2 diabetes can lead to a lot of other health problems. The symptoms of undiagnosed type 2 diabetes can be missed if you do not know what you are looking for. Or perhaps the symptoms are simply excused for some other reason ('getting older' is a common reason). Worryingly, this can go on for up to ten years, which, of course, is a serious problem.

Whilst very important, I do not want to dwell on the symptoms of undiagnosed type 2 diabetes at this point, as I will take you through those in a little while. Instead, let us take a moment to understand why type 2 diabetes should be taken seriously, and the harm it can cause to the body.

Cardiovascular disease
Cardiovascular disease includes several conditions that can affect the heart and blood vessels. Sustained high blood sugar levels can lead to the hardening or narrowing of the blood vessels, which increases the risk of heart attacks, strokes and other heart-related issues.

Diabetic Neuropathy (nerve damage)

Diabetic Neuropathy causes damage to the nerves - particularly those in the feet and hands - because of prolonged high blood sugar levels. Symptoms can range from numbness and tingling, to sharp pains that often worsen at night.

Diabetic Nephropathy (kidney damage)

Diabetic Nephropathy damages the tiny blood vessels in the kidneys, hindering their ability to effectively filter waste from the blood. Over time, it may lead to kidney failure, then dialysis or a kidney transplant.

Diabetic Retinopathy (eye damage)

Diabetic Retinopathy comes from damage to the blood vessels in the retina. It can cause blurred vision, floaters and, in severe cases, blindness.

Foot complications

Type 2 diabetes can lead to poor circulation and nerve damage in the feet, making the feet more susceptible to infections, ulcers and injuries. In extreme cases, this can also lead to foot and lower limb amputation.

Hearing impairments

Type 2 diabetes can increase the risk of hearing loss, due to damage to the blood vessels and nerves within the inner ear.

Skin disorders

Type 2 diabetes can cause skin issues, including bacterial and fungal infections, dryness, itchiness and discolouration.

Alzheimer's disease

Studies have shown a connection between type 2 diabetes and an increased risk of Alzheimer's disease - possibly because of how the disease affects blood vessels and insulin usage in the brain (though research, at the time of writing, is still ongoing).

From personal experience and that of my clients, I can tell you that with lifestyle changes (especially dietary modifications and increased physical activity) you can not only manage type 2 diabetes better but potentially reverse it too! This does not necessarily signify a 'cure' as such, but rather achieving and maintaining blood sugar levels within the normal range with no medication. And surely, that has to be a great goal to aim for!

If you are not yet diagnosed with type 2 diabetes but suspect that you might be heading down that slippery slope (or perhaps you are pre-diabetic), you too can turn things around if you choose to.

Busting Some Type 2 Diabetes Myths

You now have a basic knowledge of what type 2 diabetes is and have an understanding of the health complications related to it. So, in order to further build on your understanding of the disease, I would like to debunk some of the more common myths that I have encountered over the years.

Myth: It is the less-serious type of diabetes
Fact: All forms of diabetes are serious and can have life-altering consequences if blood sugar levels are not properly regulated.

Myth: You cannot eat any sugar
Fact: It is not about complete avoidance of sugar, but educating yourself in simple but effective methods of management, and understanding what that sugar does to your body - working towards a situation where you do not crave sugar and therefore consume less.

Myth: Type 2 diabetes is a "sugar disease"
Fact: While managing blood sugar is important for those with type 2 diabetes, to call it a "sugar disease" is to miss the point. The way sugar affects the body goes beyond the amount consumed and involves insulin's role, insulin resistance, and pancreatic function. As I have mentioned, the root causes of type 2 diabetes often run deeper and originate from more than one source.

Myth: Only overweight or obese individuals get type 2 diabetes

Fact: There is no easy way to say this - obesity is a significant risk factor when it comes to the development of type 2 diabetes, but we also know that it is not the sole determinant. Many people diagnosed are of average weight and, equally, some obese people never develop it. Diet, lifestyle, age, habits, and ethnicity are other contributors to the development of the disease. It is of note, however, that abdominal obesity (characterised by excessive visceral fat around organs and manifesting as "love handles" or the "spare tyre") presents a higher risk. This visceral fat is dangerous, as it interferes with the body's hormonal functions and increases insulin resistance, leading to elevated blood sugar levels.

Myth: Eating too much sugar causes type 2 diabetes

Fact: The direct link between sugar intake and type 2 diabetes is not always straightforward. Consuming large amounts of sugary foods and drinks can lead to weight gain, which increases the risk of developing the disease. Whilst its progression is more associated with diet and lifestyle, age and family history can sometimes be factors. Diabetic or not, cutting back on sugary drinks and snacks is beneficial.

Myth: Insulin therapy is only for severe cases of type 2 diabetes

Fact: Insulin therapy is tailored by a doctor based on an individual's needs. For some, it might be introduced early, while for others, it could be recommended later. It is not a reflection of disease severity, but is simply another tool to manage blood sugar effectively, where perhaps other medication is not effective.

Myth: People with type 2 diabetes should follow a special 'diabetic diet'

Fact: The best diet for someone with type 2 diabetes is a balanced, healthy diet. It prioritises whole natural foods, minimises processed foods, focuses on complex carbohydrates, lean proteins, healthy fats, and plenty of vegetables.

As noted in my introduction, I am not a fan of so-called 'Diets' as companies often employ them to get you to buy their products, they can be expensive and they are frequently unsustainable. All you need to be healthy and avoid (or potentially reverse) type 2 diabetes can be found in the natural foods around you.

Myth: Once on medication, dietary and lifestyle changes are secondary

Fact: Medication, including insulin and other oral medication, are simply management tools and not cures (recall my illustration of 'painting the leaves green'). Relying solely on them while ignoring diet and physical activity is a flawed strategy. Regular exercise, for example, can increase insulin sensitivity, so your body requires less insulin to process glucose. The synergy between medication, diet and lifestyle is the cornerstone of effective blood sugar control.

Myth: If you have type 2 diabetes, exercise is dangerous

Fact: On the contrary, exercise can be an effective tool in type 2 diabetes prevention and reversal. Regular physical activity can improve insulin sensitivity, reduce cardiovascular risks and aid weight loss. The key is starting slow, finding exercises you enjoy, monitoring blood sugars where appropriate and ensuring activities align with your health goals. From walking and swimming to resistance training, there are many types of exercise to enjoy that can fit in with your personal capabilities, limitations and lifestyle.

Myth: Type 2 diabetes does not present serious health risks if you feel fine

Fact: The absence of obvious symptoms does not equate to absence of disease. Chronic high blood sugar, even without noticeable symptoms, can damage blood vessels, nerves and organs. In fact, type 2 diabetes can, sometimes, take up to ten years be diagnosed – and this diagnosis often happens when either the individual notices symptoms in themselves that seem out of the ordinary, or it is picked up on a random blood test. Regular check-ups, monitoring and recognising the symptoms (which we will cover next) can lead to timely interventions.

Myth: you will know you have type 2 diabetes from the symptoms

Fact: As previously noted, many individuals with type 2 diabetes may not show obvious symptoms, especially in the early stages. It is frequently detected during routine medical examinations. Regular health check-ups are vital, even more so once you reach 40 and beyond.

Myth: Fruit is a no-go if you have type 2 diabetes

Fact: While fruits have natural sugars, they are rich in essential nutrients and fibres. Whole fruits, in moderation, are better for you than fruit juice or dried fruit.

Myth: You cannot eat carbohydrates if you have type 2 diabetes
Fact: Carbohydrates are pivotal for energy. A balanced diet consisting of all the macronutrients, together with monitoring portion sizes, is preferable to complete abstinence. Often, eliminating major food groups (like carbohydrates, for example) can cause other health issues. It is all about balance, not elimination.

Myth: Type 2 diabetes is not that serious
Fact: If improperly controlled, type 2 diabetes can lead to complications like heart disease or kidney damage as we covered in the previous section. Proper management and working towards reversal can substantially reduce these risks.

Myth: Only older adults get type 2 diabetes
Fact: Type 2 diabetes is frequently now being seen in younger adults and children, primarily because of increasing obesity rates, poor diets, sedentary lifestyles and a lack of nutritional knowledge.

Myth: Those with type 2 diabetes should avoid alcohol
Fact: While alcohol can (and often does) impact blood sugar levels, moderate consumption might be acceptable for type 2 diabetics.

Myth: People with type 2 diabetes are more prone to common illnesses
Fact: Those with type 2 diabetes do not have a heightened risk for common ailments, but illnesses can cause blood sugars to rise.

Ignorance Is Not Bliss

Often referred to as the 'silent epidemic', pre-diabetes and type 2 diabetes quietly affects hundreds of millions of people worldwide. Many are going about their daily lives completely unaware of the damage the disease is doing inside them - because they are missing the symptoms or mistaking them for something else.

I cannot stress highly enough the importance of detecting pre-diabetes or type 2 diabetes at the earliest opportunity.

With detection, a diagnosis and the right support, you can make informed lifestyle choices and adopt a sustainable diet beneficial for blood sugar control. You can do this yourself with the knowledge from books like this, or you could choose to work collaboratively with a nutritionist that specialises in helping people with pre-diabetes and type 2 diabetes.

So, let us review some symptoms to look out for…

Spotting The Symptoms

One of the major concerns regarding uncontrolled or unmonitored blood sugar is the silent progression of type 2 diabetes. Unlike some other conditions which manifest with clearly obvious symptoms from the start, type 2 diabetes can quietly develop - presenting little to no noticeable signs until significant damage has already been done. By the time symptoms like excessive thirst, fatigue, or blurred vision become apparent, the body may have been grappling with elevated blood sugar levels for many years.

There are people who (1) are not yet type 2 diabetic but who have a lifestyle that is leading them down that pathway, (2) are knowingly or unknowingly are pre-diabetic (that is, those with higher than normal blood sugar levels but not yet in the 'diabetic range'), (3) are living with type 2 diabetes who are diagnosed and likely on medication and (4) have type 2 diabetes, but are completely unaware of the fact.

This section is for people in categories (2) and (4) - those who are pre-diabetic or type 2 diabetic but not yet diagnosed and are therefore unaware of the damage happening inside them.

"But", I hear you ask, "how do I know if I have type 2 diabetes without having to go to my doctor"?

Type 2 diabetes leaves a trail to follow, and if you know what you are looking for, then spotting the symptoms can be remarkably easy.

It is important to note that some people with type 2 diabetes may not experience any symptoms, especially in the early stages and regular check-ups (and blood tests) can help to catch the disease early, even in the absence of noticeable symptoms.

Remember... If in doubt, get it checked out!

(Note: you may relate to one or more of these symptoms and it may concern you. Recognising these symptoms does not mean you have type 2 diabetes. That said, I encourage you to pay a visit to your doctor for a blood glucose check - particularly if you have not had one done in the last few years).

The Symptoms of High Blood Sugars

Frequent urination (Polyuria)
Many with undiagnosed type 2 diabetes experience an increased need to urinate and a telltale sign is the need to get up in the night regularly for bathroom visits. This is one of the biggest signs and one that should never be ignored.
What to look for: Going to the toilet more frequently, especially at night.

Increased thirst (Polydipsia)

As the body tries to offset the fluid lost through frequent urination, you may feel thirstier than usual. This is an unusual type of thirst, as it is not satisfied no matter how much water is consumed.

What to look for: Continually reaching for a drink and not feeling satisfied after drinking.

Unintended weight loss

Despite eating 'as normal' (or indeed perhaps eating more than normal), rapid and unexplained weight loss can be a concern. The body, starved of energy from glucose, starts breaking down muscle and fat for fuel. This can lead to unexpected losses in weight.

What to look for: Sudden or gradual weight loss, despite not trying to lose weight or possibly eating more.

Persistent fatigue (Asthenia)

Insufficient glucose reaching the body's cells can leave you constantly feeling fatigued or exhausted.

What to look for: Feeling weary, needing to rest more often, struggling to get through the day.

Increased hunger (Polyphagia)

Closely linked to fatigue and overeating, when the body cannot use glucose as a fuel source it demands more food, leading to constant hunger, known as Polyphagia.

What to look for: Eating more than usual, but still feeling hungry.

Blurred vision

High blood sugar levels can cause fluid to be pulled from the lenses of the eyes, leading to blurred vision. Over time, type 2 diabetes can cause new blood vessels to form in the retina and damage established vessels.
What to look for: Difficulty reading, recognising faces, or seeing things in focus. Intermittent blurred vision.

Slow healing of cuts and wounds

Elevated blood sugar affects the body's ability to heal. Blood flow may be impaired and infections can occur more easily. A minor cut or bruise may take weeks to heal, making the skin more susceptible to infections.
What to look for: Sores, ulcers or cuts that take weeks or months to heal.

Frequent infections

Type 2 diabetes can weaken the immune system, making the body less able to fight off infections. Common places for these infections to occur are the bladder, kidneys, skin, and gums.
What to look for: Recurring skin infections, urinary tract infections, or respiratory infections.

Frequent urinary tract infections (UTIs)

Type 2 diabetics are at a higher risk because of impaired immune function and elevated blood sugar levels.
What to look for: Burning sensation during urination, cloudy or blood-tinged urine, a frequent urge to urinate.

Recurrent yeast infections (Candidiasis)

Excess sugar in the blood and urine provides food for yeast, leading to infections.

What to look for: Persistent fungal infections on the skin, mouth (oral thrush), or genital areas.

Tingling or numbness (Peripheral Neuropathy)

Peripheral Neuropathy (nerve damage) manifests as tingling, numbness or pain in the hands and feet caused by prolonged exposure to high blood sugar affecting delicate nerve fibres.

What to look for: A frequent sensation of "pins and needles", coldness, or numbness, particularly in the extremities.

Itchy skin (Pruritus)

Excess sugar in the blood and urine can be a feeding ground for bacteria and yeast, leading to infections. Such infections can present as itchy rashes, commonly in moist areas like the armpits or groin.

What to look for: Persistent itching, often with visible skin rashes or dryness.

Dry skin (Xerosis)

Type 2 diabetes can cause dehydration, leading to dry skin.

What to look for: Cracked, flaky, or rough skin, especially on the legs and feet.

Darkened skin patches (Acanthosis Nigricans)

Acanthosis Nigricans is a condition where dark, velvety patches appear in body creases and folds.

What to look for: Dark, velvety patches, typically on the neck, armpits, or groin.

Presence of areas of darkened skin (Hyperpigmentation)

Similar to Acanthosis Nigricans, patches of darkened skin indicate insulin resistance or hormonal imbalances.

What to look for: Dark patches on skin, often symmetrically on both sides of the body.

Feeling irritable

Fluctuating blood sugars can lead to mood swings and irritability.

What to look for: Quick mood changes, lower tolerance to stress, snapping at minor annoyances.

Gum infections (Gingivitis or Periodontitis)

Diabetes reduces the body's ability to fight bacteria, increasing the risk for gum infections.

What to look for: Red, swollen, or bleeding gums, persistent bad breath.

I know I sound like a broken record, but it is just so important to recognise the early symptoms of type 2 diabetes. If you can relate to any of these symptoms and it worries you, please get it checked out, especially if you haven't had a HBA1C check in the past 18-24 months.

Maybe your symptoms are nothing to be concerned about, but perhaps they are. Checking your blood glucose will remove doubt and allow you to take action if there is an issue.

Remember, ignorance is <u>not</u> bliss.

Step 1: Nutrition

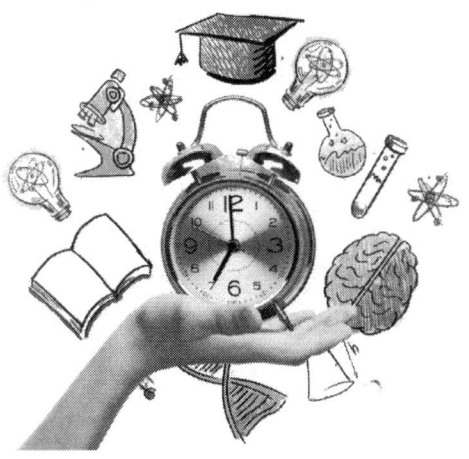

Introduction

I would like to take you back to nutritional basics. From my personal experience (and of working with clients who begin their type 2 diabetes journey with no background in nutrition), the foundation of lasting change is knowledge. Knowledge brings understanding, and the power to make better choices.

Knowledge is the important first step of The KISSS Plan, as knowledge (or, to be more precise, applied knowledge) can be powerful. A basic understanding of nutrition - specifically nutrition that relates to blood sugar control - can help you too. You will make smarter choices and will not be just following instructions without knowing the real reasons why. You will understand the logic, the thinking, and the rationale behind the actions you take.

If you have little understanding of the basics of nutrition, step 1 will really help you. I won't delve too deeply into each subject, as it's unnecessary to make things overly complicated. Plus, there are other books available that provide more in-depth research on each subject. I would prefer to give you an overview of each subject to pique your interest and to give you enough information to make sense of it, and to take action.

If you have a basic understanding of nutrition, it might tempt you to skip step 1 and move on to step 2 – and I would encourage you not to do that. I am constantly learning more and more each day about nutrition; it is an almost endless subject. I would take a guess and say that even if you have a reasonable knowledge of nutrition, there is always scope to learn more.

So, on that note, let us dive in.

The Journey of Glucose: From Plate to Cell

At the heart of your body's energy system is a simple sugar called glucose. Glucose is vital to life as, without it, your body would lack the essential fuel needed to carry out even the most basic tasks. Glucose powers largely everything you do. It is your body's preferred source of energy.

One of the most incredible processes within your body is how you transform the food you eat into the energy you need to survive. The process of digestion is one that is rarely given a second thought by many people. The food goes in your mouth. You chew. You taste. You swallow… and then what?

What happens next and why should you care?

Well, in relation to blood sugar control, a basic understanding of the digestive process is important.

Let me give you an illustration. You own a factory, and on the assembly line each worker has a specific task that ensures the final product is created correctly and to specification. As the business owner, it would make sense to have at least a basic understanding of what is going on in your factory, to ensure the production line works effectively, and that your factory is producing the end product as it should be. In a similar way, your digestive system is a complex factory with many moving parts that all work with each other, and having a basic understanding of the process can help you maximise its effectiveness.

The moment food enters your mouth and you chew, you are not just mechanically breaking down your food (although chewing is very important and helps with satiety) - chewing also kick-starts the chemical process of breaking carbohydrates down.

Simple sugars require minimal breakdown and are rapidly absorbed into the bloodstream. Complex carbohydrates take longer, as they first need to be broken down into simpler sugars (primarily glucose) before absorption. In the stomach, enzymes produced both by the intestinal lining and the pancreas get to work, breaking down the food into its component parts. Simple sugars, including glucose, are then absorbed through the intestinal walls and enter the bloodstream, leading to an increase in blood sugar levels.

It is important to understand that not all carbohydrates are created equal, as their structure and composition can significantly influence how quickly they are converted into glucose. For example, whole grains (which contain a higher fibre content) are broken down and absorbed more slowly than refined grains, leading to more gradual rises in blood sugar levels.

While carbohydrates are the primary contributors to blood glucose, they are not the only ones. In situations where carbohydrate intake is low (such as in certain diets or prolonged fasting), your body can produce glucose from non-carbohydrate sources, where proteins and fats can be converted too (a process called gluconeogenesis).

Maintaining balanced blood sugar levels is crucial in preventing and reversing type 2 diabetes. A diet that leads to rapid and regular spikes in blood sugar can put pressure on the body's insulin response mechanism, which can lead to insulin resistance.

Insulin and Blood Sugar Control

Insulin, a hormone produced by the pancreas (a glandular organ nestled deep within the abdomen and neighbour to the liver), is a key player in blood sugar control. Whenever you eat carbohydrates, your digestive system breaks these down into simple sugars (primarily glucose) and as the glucose enters your bloodstream, it signals to the pancreas to release insulin. But what exactly does insulin do?

Think of it this way: body cells have doors that can be unlocked to allow glucose through and to be used for energy. Insulin is the key that unlocks these doors. When the insulin key no longer properly fits the lock, glucose cannot enter the cells, and it remains in the bloodstream.

If left unchecked, higher than normal blood sugar levels can cause damage to the body. Insulin's job is to bring glucose into cells for energy and safeguard against high blood sugar damage.

You may have previously heard of the terms 'insulin sensitivity' and 'insulin resistance'. Insulin sensitivity describes how receptive your cells are to insulin itself as, when the cells are sensitive, only a small amount of insulin is required to open cell doors and let glucose in.

On the other hand, insulin resistance means that the cells are not responding as they should to insulin, becoming 'resistant' to its effect. As a result, the pancreas then tries to produce more insulin to compensate and, over time, these persistently high levels of insulin can exhaust the pancreas as it tries to keep up with the increasing demands.

In type 2 diabetes, either not enough insulin is being is being produced, or the cells are not responding to it properly. Whatever the cause, the outcome is the same: blood sugar levels that remain higher than they should be, and for much longer than is ideal.

The Sugar Addiction Cycle

Sugar can give us a buzz, make us feel temporarily 'good', is celebrated and accepted as a reward system for children and adults alike, and is used as a coping mechanism by some when they are stressed or sad.

But let us not ignore the fact that sugar is a legal drug, and it does incredible amounts of damage to our bodies, to our families and to society.

The regular use of sugar can become a recurring cycle, known as the 'sugar addiction cycle'. Understanding this cycle is important in being able to break its grip - especially when you are focused on preventing or reversing type 2 diabetes.

As you read through the stages of the cycle, you may recognise the pattern in your own dietary habits - and that is ok. Once you understand how the sugar addiction cycle works, you can look at ways to overcome it and beat the habit.

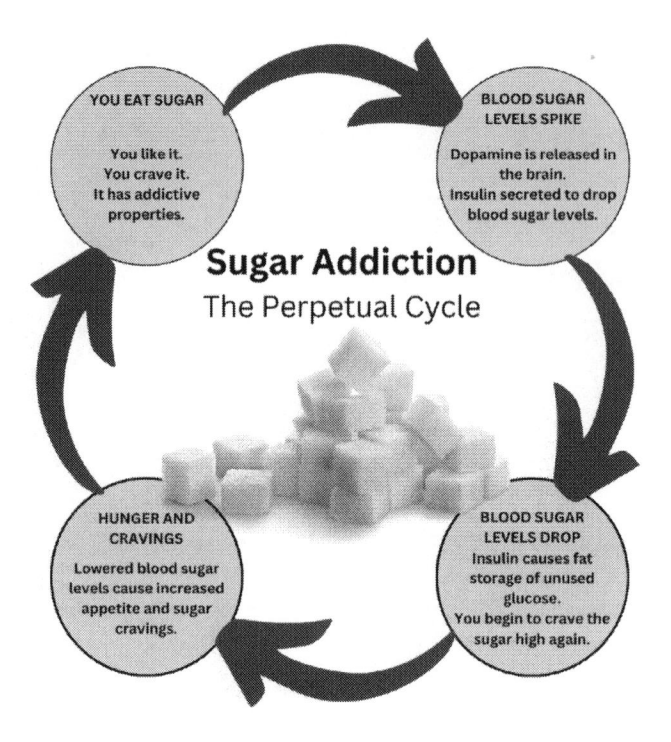

Sugar Addiction
The Perpetual Cycle

YOU EAT SUGAR
You like it.
You crave it.
It has addictive properties.

BLOOD SUGAR LEVELS SPIKE
Dopamine is released in the brain.
Insulin secreted to drop blood sugar levels.

BLOOD SUGAR LEVELS DROP
Insulin causes fat storage of unused glucose.
You begin to crave the sugar high again.

HUNGER AND CRAVINGS
Lowered blood sugar levels cause increased appetite and sugar cravings.

The temptation: Consuming sugar

When you indulge in that piece of cake or sip on a sweetened drink, sugar enters your body. The choice to consume the sugar in the first place can be driven by several factors, from its pleasant taste, its ability to offer instant energy, the comfort you feel it can bring, or even cheering you up if you are feeling down.

Pleasure and reward: Dopamine release

As you consume sugar, your brain's reward system is activated, which releases dopamine (a neurotransmitter responsible for our feelings of pleasure and satisfaction). Like many drugs, our bodies can become tolerant of sugar over time, making us crave more.

Blood sugar rises: The spike

After we consume sugar, it is broken down in our body and then enters the bloodstream, resulting in increased blood sugar levels. The body, always striving for balance (homeostasis), recognises this spike and then acts to regulate it.

Insulin jumps into action: The balancing act

As we learnt in the previous section, insulin is the body's primary blood sugar regulator, and it is secreted in response to the rising blood sugar levels. Insulin's job is essential to our health and wellbeing: it helps our cells take in the glucose from the bloodstream to be used for energy.

From spike to dip: Blood sugar levels drop

By encouraging our cells to take in and make use of the glucose in our blood, blood sugar levels drop back down again. However, insulin can be a double-edged sword and it plays two key roles once in the bloodstream - glucose uptake and fat storage. Any glucose that is not immediately needed (or cannot be utilised, as with insulin resistance) for energy by the body cells then gets stored as fat.

The aftermath: Cravings and increased appetite

After the drop in blood sugar levels, the body craves that initial sugar high that was driven by the dopamine-induced pleasure. Lowered blood sugar levels can also trigger sensations of hunger, which then encourages to you to seek more food – often sugary food – to satisfy this hunger. This can lead to overeating and weight gain.

Back to square one: The cycle continues

With the cravings and increased appetite, we often then reach for something sweet again. And so the cycle then continues - sugar consumption, dopamine release, blood sugar spike, insulin action, blood sugar drop, cravings and back to consumption.

The first step in overcoming sugar addiction is recognising its stages and being aware of its impact on you.

>> ACTION POINTS - PRIORITY 1 <<

Stay hydrated: Aim to drink at least 8 glasses (2 litres) of water a day and monitor how this impacts your sugar cravings

Start by keeping a reusable water bottle with you throughout the day. This visual cue reminds you to take sips often. Aim to refill it regularly, track your consumption towards the 2-litre goal and as you drink more water, observe any changes that you feel with your sugar cravings. Sometimes we confuse thirst with hunger, leading to unnecessary snacking.

Mindful eating: Before reaching for a sugary snack, pause for a moment

The next time you are tempted by a sugary treat, pause and take a deep breath. Reflect on what is driving that desire. Is it true hunger or an emotional need? If it is an emotional need, then think of what might really help you are that moment in time - perhaps a short walk, a cup of herbal tea, or even a quick chat with a friend. By pausing to recognise and understand your cravings and then taking action to distract yourself from those craving, you can slowly rewire our habits.

Start small: Often, reducing sugar consumption little by little over weeks or sometimes months can make weaning you off sugar easier

Begin by identifying one sugary item in your daily diet. Maybe it is that afternoon chocolate bar or your morning latte. Next, consider a slight modification: choose a small amount of dark chocolate with less sugar or reduce the sugar in your coffee. Gradually extend this practice to other foods and drinks over a few weeks, celebrating small victories along the way. This incremental approach not only makes the process more manageable but also supports a sustainable shift towards better blood sugar control.

>> ACTION POINTS - PRIORITY 2 <<

Educate yourself: Spend a day reading food labels during your grocery shopping

While shopping, take the time to read the nutritional information on the back of products. Note the sugar content, especially in foods you frequently buy, and if the sugar seems high, jot it down on a separate list. At home, take a moment to explore online to discover healthier alternatives with less sugar. Simply being aware can help you avoid hidden sugars and make smarter food choices.

Maintain a food diary: For a week, jot down everything you consume

Choose a dedicated notebook or a mobile app specifically designed for tracking food intake and then throughout the day, quickly note down everything you consume, no matter how small. At the end of the day, take a few moments to review your entries, highlighting foods and drinks that are high in sugar. Then reflect upon situations or emotions that triggered a craving for sugary items. Over time, this simple habit will offer insights into your sugar consumption patterns and help you make more informed dietary choices.

The Balancing Act

Maintaining balanced blood sugar levels is essential for good health, and we looked earlier at the complications that can occur when those levels are allowed to be left too high for too long. Imbalances in blood sugar levels are called as hypoglycaemia (too low) and hyperglycaemia (too high). Whilst low blood sugars can be a complication related to type 2 diabetes, high blood sugar is a far more common problem.

High blood sugar: Hyperglycaemia
When you consume large amounts of sugar or simple carbohydrates, you overload your system, making the pancreas work overtime. If your body cannot efficiently use the glucose due to the sheer volume of carbohydrates or other factors such as insulin resistance, blood sugar levels can spike and subsequently stay high for long periods of time.

Low blood sugar: Hypoglycaemia
Whilst we rarely associate hypoglycaemia with type 2 diabetes in the same way that we do hyperglycaemia, it can be of equal concern. Various scenarios can trigger hypoglycaemia, including regularly skipping meals, excessive alcohol consumption or an imbalance in medication. Type 2 diabetics can experience hypoglycaemic episodes, particularly if their glucose-lowering medications are not adjusted according to their diet or activity levels.

Achieving balance

Achieving blood sugar balance is the goal, and regular blood glucose monitoring (together with a balanced diet that is low in refined sugars and high in fibre) can help maintain stable blood sugar levels. Exercising regularly not only helps the body use glucose for energy, but can also increase insulin sensitivity too, helping to reduce resistance. It is also good to keep a healthy weight, as this can further reduce the risk.

If you are already diagnosed, it is never too late. With conscious and sustained dietary changes together with the committed application of the relevant action points in this book, you will probably see a significant improvement in your blood sugar levels and overall health, and have the genuine prospect of reversing your type 2 diabetes.

The Macronutrients

At the most basic level, the food you eat can be categorised as a carbohydrate, a protein, or a fat - and each has a unique role in the body. In the upcoming sections, we will discuss all three macronutrients. However, for our discussion on glucose and type 2 diabetes, carbohydrates play the key role.

Carbohydrates

When looking at our diet, carbohydrates often attract the most attention - especially in relation to type 2 diabetes. They play an important role in your energy dynamics and, if consumed in regularly and in excess, can negatively affect your blood sugar levels.

The quality of the carbohydrates you consume influences how your body processes and uses them. Compared to simple carbohydrates, complex carbohydrates are digested slower and provide a steadier release of glucose. This helps to prevent rapid spikes and crashes in blood sugar levels.

While quality is important, the quantity cannot be ignored as over-consumption of even the highest quality carbohydrates can have detrimental effects on your health. Consuming large amounts of carbohydrates (regardless of their type) can cause excessive glucose entering the bloodstream, and lead to a caloric surplus. This surplus can lead to weight gain, which can put a further strain on the body.

Simple carbohydrates
These simple sugars are basic units of carbohydrates and are termed 'simple' because of their chemical structure - which is typically made up of one or two sugar molecules. This structure allows them to be easily and rapidly absorbed by your body, and often result in a quick surge of

energy. However, this rapid absorption can lead to spikes in blood sugar levels, especially if these sugars are consumed with no accompaniments like fibre, fat or protein.

Sugar plays a pivotal role in the development and progression of type 2 diabetes. It is irresistibly sweet and comforting, and can trap us in the sugar addiction cycle. While sugar itself is not inherently 'bad', our modern diets are full of added and processed sugars. This has led to excessive sugar consumption (especially in the form of extremely damaging high-fructose corn syrup (HFCS)) across the world, and the subsequent type 2 diabetes health crisis that we are now witnessing.

Simple sugars are broadly categorised in to two different types - Monosaccharides and Disaccharides, and it would be useful for you to have a basic overview of each:

Monosaccharides

These are the basic single molecules of carbohydrates. Glucose is the body's primary energy source), but there are two other types too:

- Fructose: Mainly found in fruits, honey, and root vegetables. While fructose naturally occurs in fruits, it is also a component of the highly controversial high-fructose corn syrup (we will discuss fruit and fructose in more detail later in the book).
- Galactose: Rarely found on its own, galactose is normally found bound to glucose to form lactose.

Disaccharides

These comprise two monosaccharides stuck together with a weak chemical bond, and there are three types:
- Sucrose (glucose + fructose): White table sugar, found naturally in many plants.
- Lactose (glucose + galactose): Found in milk and dairy products.
- Maltose (glucose + glucose): Malt sugar that is found in certain grains, and is produced during the malting process.

Monosaccharides and disaccharides are quickly digested and absorbed into the bloodstream. However, not all simple carbohydrates are a problem (for instance, the fructose in whole fruits comes bundled with fibre and other nutrients, which slows the speed of the sugar's absorption and mitigates its impact on blood sugar).

Simple sugars are everywhere in our food - they are not just in sweets, soft drinks and added to most processed foods (often for taste and/or as a preservative), but are also found in natural foods too:
- Fruits: While fruits contain fructose, they are also packed with essential vitamins, minerals, fibres, and antioxidants.
- Dairy products: As mentioned, lactose is the primary sugar in milk and other dairy products. However, lactose is metabolised differently than other simple sugars and rarely leads to rapid spikes in blood sugar (but still needs to be accounted for in your daily total sugar intake).

Sugar's allure can be tempting, but the dangers it poses in relation to type 2 diabetes and its progression are undeniable. Be assured that by arming yourself with knowledge and making conscious choices to limit your sugar intake, you can take control of your health.

Please download my handy "sugar names" pocket guide, at **www.diabetessolutions.co.uk/tkp-bonuspack**

Complex carbohydrates

Complex carbohydrates have a more 'complex' molecular structure (hence their name). This means that they are digested slower and release their energy more gradually, which results in much less pronounced blood sugar spikes.

Complex carbohydrates are found in natural and unprocessed foods, and they come packed with vitamins, minerals, dietary fibre and more that are essential to our good health. These nutrients help with supporting digestion, improving immune function, stabilising blood sugars, promoting a healthy gut microbiome, and reducing the risk of cancer.

We do not need to get too technical on the topic of complex carbohydrates, but it is useful to know a little about the two different groups:

Oligosaccharides ('oligo' means 'few')

Oligosaccharides have chains that contain between three and ten glucose molecules each, and can be categorised in to three subgroups:

- Fructo-oligosaccharides (FOS): These are found in various fruits and vegetables, including bananas, onions, and garlic.
- Galacto-oligosaccharides (GOS): These are found in legumes and certain dairy products.
- Human Milk Oligosaccharides (HMOs): These are naturally present in human breast milk.

Polysaccharides ('poly' means 'many')

Polysaccharides have chains that contain ten or more glucose molecules. They are categorised into three primary sub-groups:

- Starches: These are the principal storage form of energy in plants and comprise many glucose units (as opposed to simple carbohydrates that have just one or two). Common sources include grains, legumes and tubers. Your body breaks down starches into glucose over a longer period compared to simple carbohydrates, providing a more sustained energy release and with less risk of blood sugar spikes.
- Dietary fibres (cellulose): Unlike other carbohydrates, fibre is not digested by the body. Found mainly in plant foods, fibre is essential for your digestive health. While your body does not absorb fibre in the same way it does with other nutrients, fibre aids in promoting healthy digestion and keeping your gut in good condition. Dietary fibre can be soluble (dissolves in water) or insoluble (does not dissolve). Soluble fibre can help manage blood sugar levels by slowing the absorption of sugar. Good sources of fibre include vegetables, fruit, oats, beans, and whole grains. We will cover fibre as a separate topic shortly.

- Glycogen: Think of glycogen as your body's energy reserve. It is the way your body stocks up on extra glucose for use later, mainly in your liver and muscles and each glycogen molecule can have up to 50,000 glucose molecules in a single chain. Glycogen can also provide rapid energy during short-term, intense activities.

Foods that are high in complex carbohydrates typically come with other vital nutrients and given their structure and fibre content, they are more filling. This can help regulate appetite and possibly help with weight management.

The misunderstanding around fruits
Fruit, given its fructose content, is sometimes mistakenly seen as 'bad' for blood sugar. However, fruit offers a range of health benefits, and you should not be dissuaded from eating it in moderation. We will cover fruits in a separate section later.

>> ACTION POINTS - PRIORITY 1 <<

Assess your sugar intake: Begin by evaluating your current sugar consumption. I cannot stress how critical this action point is, consider it non-negotiable! This really is the first step in the prevention or reversal of type 2 diabetes.

*Assess your refined sugar intake by keeping an online food diary for a week or two. Note down **EVERYTHING** you eat and drink, including* *meals, snacks, and drinks. Be thorough and honest in recording your choices, and pay special attention to sources of added or refined sugars that come from sugary drinks, sweets, and processed foods (do not include fruit when eaten in its natural form in this total - but if you eat fruit, please do so in moderation). This self-awareness exercise will reveal your sugar consumption patterns and help you make informed decisions to reduce your intake.*

Set yourself an absolute daily added sugar intake limit, and over the coming weeks work towards the target of no more than 20g per day (remember, this 20g limit relates to refined and processed sugars - i.e. those foods/drinks that come from a factory, are not found in nature, have been processed in some way, and generally come in tins, packets and boxes). Vegetables, and moderate consumption of fruit, are excluded from this limit.

*In addition, in conjunction with an online food diary app, try to keep your **MAXIMUM** daily net carbohydrates (that is, total carbohydrates minus fibre) to **no more than 100-120g per day**, and **no more than 40-50g per meal**.*

Read food labels: Learn to read food labels and spot hidden sugars
Start by picking up items you commonly consume at the shops and look at the nutrition label. Pay close attention to the 'carbohydrates' section, where 'sugars' are listed. Scan for various sugar names such as high-fructose corn syrup (HFCS), agave nectar, or maltose (keep my pocket guide with you and refer to it). Keep in mind that ingredients are

usually listed in descending order of quantity, so if sugar (or a sugar alias) appears near the top, treat it as a red flag. By regularly practicing this skill, you'll quickly become proficient in spotting hidden sugars and making informed choices.

Reduce sugary foods: Gradually reduce your intake of sugary snacks, fizzy drinks, and processed foods
Transitioning to a lower-sugar diet can be achieved step by step by identifying one sugary food or drink in your daily routine that you can easily replace. For instance, if you regularly have a sugary drink with your lunch, swap it for sparkling water. Then gradually substitute other sugary snacks with whole foods like fruits, nuts, or Greek yogurt. If you need a little sweetness, opt for natural alternatives like honey or maple syrup (but in strict moderation).

Choose balanced meals: Prioritise balanced meals rich in vegetables, lean proteins, and whole grains
Fill half your plate with non-starchy vegetables (like leafy greens, broccoli, or peppers), then add a palm-sized portion of lean protein (such as chicken, fish or tofu), then complete your plate with a serving of whole grains (like brown rice or quinoa). This technique helps stabilise blood sugars by slowing the absorption of carbohydrates.

Stay Active: Incorporate regular movement or exercise into your daily routine
Incorporating regular physical activity into your daily routine can be straightforward. We will cover movement and exercise in step 2.

>> ACTION POINT - PRIORITY 2 <<

Regular monitoring: If you have type 2 diabetes, regularly monitor your blood sugar levels as advised by your doctor

Regular monitoring of your blood sugar levels is an important part of controlling blood sugars effectively. Start by consulting your doctor to determine the recommended frequency and times for checking your blood sugar (or perhaps invest in a constant glucose monitoring machine to avoid the need for regular finger-pricking).

Make it a daily routine (perhaps 2 hours after each meal) to track how your readings respond to different foods. Keep a log or use a mobile app to record your results and discuss your readings with your doctor. The act of consistently monitoring your blood sugar will help you gain insight into how well you are controlling your blood sugar, and will help you make informed decisions about your diet.

Sugar By Any Other Name

When trying to reduce the amount of sugar you consume, looking out for 'sugar' on food labels makes sense. Once upon a time, it was easy to spot 'sugar' on packaging. These days, identifying sugar and its derivatives on food labels can be challenging because they are hidden under many different names.

I have listed below the more common names for sugar in food, and where they can commonly be found (there are even more than are listed below, over 60 at the last count!). You do not need to remember these, but I hope that by bringing them to your attention, it might just help you pick them out the next time you look at a food label.

As a rule of thumb, any syrup or any substance ending in 'ose' will be a sugar of some type or another.

- **Agave nectar:** Extracted from the agave plant; often found in so-called 'health foods' as a natural sweetener.
- **Barley malt syrup:** Made from sprouted barley; used in some baked goods.
- **Brown rice syrup (and rice syrup):** Made by breaking down rice starches; found in so-called 'health food' products.

- **Brown sugar:** White sugar with molasses added; commonly used in baking.
- **Buttered syrup:** Combination of sugar and butter, used in confectionery.
- **Cane sugar:** Made from sugarcane.
- **Caramel:** Cooked sugar; used for colour and flavour in food and soft drinks.
- **Carob syrup:** Made from carob pods; found in health food products.
- **Castor sugar:** Very fine granulated sugar; used in baking.
- **Coconut sugar:** Extracted from coconut palm sap; a healthier sugar alternative.
- **Confectioner's sugar:** Finely ground sugar; used for icing.
- **Corn sweetener:** Corn-derived sweetener; found in many processed foods.
- **Corn syrup:** Made from cornflour; used in sweets and processed foods.
- **Corn syrup solids:** Dehydrated corn syrup; used in dry products.
- **Date sugar:** Made from dehydrated dates; found in natural food products.
- **Demerara sugar:** A type of raw cane sugar; used in coffee and baking.
- **Dextrin:** Hydrolysed starch; used in processed foods.
- **Dextrose:** Sugar derived from starches; common in baking and processed foods.

- **Evaporated cane juice:** Less processed cane sugar; found in some baked goods.
- **Fructose:** Sugar found in fruits; often extracted and used in abundance in drinks, sweets and processed foods.
- **Fruit juice concentrate:** Concentrated fruit sugars; used in many processed foods.
- **Galactose:** found in dairy products.
- **Glucose:** Simple sugar; used in sweets, desserts and syrups.
- **Golden sugar:** Less refined brown sugar; used in baking.
- **Golden syrup:** Refined sugar syrup; used in baking and desserts.
- **Grape sugar:** Another term for glucose.
- **High-fructose corn syrup (HFCS):** A highly controversial processed liquid sweetener; common in soft drinks.
- **Honey:** Natural sweetener from bees; used in various foods and drinks.
- **Icing sugar:** Another name for confectioner's sugar.
- **Invert sugar:** Broken down sucrose; used in confections to prevent crystallisation.
- **Lactose:** Sugar found in milk.
- **Malt syrup:** Syrup from barley malt; used in some baked goods.
- **Maltodextrin:** Starch-derived sugar; used in processed foods.
- **Maltol:** Naturally occurring sugar; used for flavour enhancement.

- **Maltose:** Sugar formed from malt; found in beers and malted foods.
- **Maple syrup:** Natural syrup from maple trees; used as a sweetener.
- **Molasses:** Sugarcane byproduct; used in baking.
- **Muscovado sugar:** Unrefined sugar with molasses; used in baked goods.
- **Raw sugar:** Less refined sugar; used as a general sweetener.
- **Refiner's syrup:** Byproduct of refining sugar; used in confectionery.
- **Saccharose:** The scientific name for sucrose; found in many sweetened products.
- **Sucrose:** Common table sugar; found in a vast array of processed foods.

So, as you can see, spotting sugars on food labels can be quite tricky!

From that list, I draw your attention to some specific sugars and sugar derivatives that have raised health concerns in recent years:

High-fructose corn syrup (HFCS)

HFCS is associated with obesity, heart disease and type 2 diabetes. The body metabolises HFCS differently to other sugars and high consumption can lead to increased fat deposits in the liver (a condition known as non-alcoholic fatty liver disease (NAFLD)), insulin resistance and other metabolic issues.

Agave nectar/syrup

Although marketed as a natural and healthier alternative to sugar, agave nectar is high in fructose (even more than HFCS, sometimes). The high fructose content can present the same metabolic issues as HFCS when consumed in large amounts.

Fructose

Pure fructose extracted from its natural source (sometimes fruit, often corn) can be a problem. Like HFCS, it is metabolised in the liver, where it can be converted into glucose but also stored as fat. Excessive fructose intake (specifically when it has been added to processed foods and drinks) can contribute to weight gain, insulin resistance, and other health issues.

Sugar alcohols (e.g. xylitol, sorbitol, maltitol)

While they provide fewer calories than traditional sugars and do not impact blood sugar levels as much, they can cause digestive upset (like gas, bloating and diarrhoea).

Artificial sweeteners

Though not sugars or derivatives, these sugar substitutes are worth mentioning. Their safety is still being debated, but some studies show potential risks like changes to gut bacteria and a paradoxical effect on glucose intolerance. We will cover artificial sweeteners a little later.

While the body prefers glucose, issues arise when carbohydrates are consumed excessively or primarily from poor dietary sources. As always, the poison is in the dose and therefore moderation is key, and prioritising whole foods over heavily processed options can help regulate total sugar intake.

Whilst diligence with identifying the sugars in your food and drink is encouraged, please do not overly stress over it – stick with it, as being able to pick out different sugar types gets easier with time and experience.

Please download my handy "sugar names" pocket guide, and make good use of it when you are next out shopping at
www.diabetessolutions.co.uk/tkp-bonuspack

Protein

Proteins are the building blocks of life, and are found in all living cells (humans, animals and even plants). They are formed from chains of twenty different amino acids, and these are linked in specific sequences (just like letters of the alphabet combine to form words and sentences). These amino acid sequences determine each protein's unique structure and function. The human body can produce eleven of these, the 'non-essential' amino acids. The remaining nine, the 'essential' amino acids, must be sourced from your diet.

Foods that provide all nine essential amino acids are considered 'complete' protein sources. These include meat, fish, eggs, and dairy. In contrast, most plant-based sources (like beans or grains) lack one or more essential amino acids and are known as 'incomplete'. However, by combining various plant foods, like nuts, seeds, beans and rice, you can get a complete protein profile.

In your body, proteins provide structure to cells and enable your organs, muscles, and tissues to maintain their integrity. They also act as enzymes that speed up chemical reactions (without enzymes, processes like digestion and energy production would occur too slowly to sustain life).

Proteins help move molecules around your body (haemoglobin, a protein found in blood, is a good example, as it carries oxygen from the lungs to other body parts). Antibodies, a type of protein, play an essential role in your immune response, defending against harmful invaders.

Some proteins function as hormones, transmitting signals between cells and coordinating bodily processes. Insulin (which we know is critical in blood sugar control) is one such protein.

We learnt from the previous section that carbohydrates are the primary influencers of your blood sugar levels, but you may not know that proteins also have an effect - albeit more subtle.

When consumed on their own, proteins have minimal immediate impact on blood sugar. However, they can influence blood sugars in the following ways:

Delayed blood sugar rise
When eaten with carbohydrates, proteins can slow the absorption of sugar, which results in a more gradual blood sugar rise.

Gluconeogenesis
In the absence of carbohydrates (such as in a zero or very low carbohydrate dies), or during periods of intense physical activity, the body can convert some amino acids into glucose through a process called gluconeogenesis.

Insulin sensitivity

Regular protein intake (especially from plant-based sources) can help to improve insulin sensitivity.

Striking a balance with protein consumption is essential. Too little protein causes muscle loss, fatigue, and weakened immune system, while too much protein, especially from animals, strains the kidneys and poses other health risks.

>> ACTION POINTS - PRIORITY 1 <<

Be label-savvy: When shopping for packaged protein sources (especially plant-based alternatives) always check the label for protein content, added sugars and other additives
Start by looking at the nutritional information and scan first for protein content to ensure you are getting a substantial amount from that product. Then look at the sugars and try to keep these to a minimum. Lastly, look at the ingredient list for any unfamiliar names and if there are additives or ingredients you cannot pronounce, reconsider your choice.

Mind your portions: Familiarise yourself with appropriate serving sizes to avoid over-consumption
When considering portion size, a practical approach is to use your hand as a guide. For proteins, aim for a piece roughly the size and thickness of your palm. This provides a personalised reference, as hand

sizes often correlate with our body size. Over time, you will intuitively know the right amount.

>> ACTION POINTS - PRIORITY 2 <<

Variety is important: Aim to incorporate different protein sources throughout the week
Start by planning your weekly meals - perhaps have two days for fish, two days for lean meats (like chicken or turkey) and reserve the remaining days for plant-based proteins (such as lentils, chickpeas, or tofu). This not only provides you with a range of essential amino acids, but also introduces varied flavours and textures.

Meal planning: As you plan your meals, focus on including a variety of protein sources (and balance them with carbohydrates and fats)
Designate certain days of the week for specific protein sources, like 'meat-free Mondays' or 'fish Fridays' and then, using a simple chart, list down each meal and ensure there is a protein presence. Alongside the protein, pencil in a small serving of whole grain carbohydrates, like quinoa or brown rice and healthy fats, such as avocados or nuts. With this visual guide, you will easily maintain variety and the chart ensures a healthy balance between the food groups, helping stabilise your blood sugar levels.

Cooking methods matter: Opt for grilling, baking, or steaming over frying to retain the lean nature of your protein source

To best preserve the nutritional value of your proteins, review your cooking methods. If you are used to frying chicken or fish, try marinating them with your favourite herbs and spices and then grilling or baking them in the oven. For vegetables or seafood, steaming is a great option as it locks in flavour without adding extra fat.

Dietary Fat

Dietary fat has been a topic of confusion for many decades, and that has led to a barrage of so-called 'healthy' low-fat and zero-fat products. Breaking down the complexities of fats into simple terms can help you make smarter food choices. Fat, from a biological perspective, consist of glycerol and fatty acids, and are dense energy sources - offering more than double the energy of proteins or carbohydrates per gram. However, fats are not just about energy; they have a range of very important functions in the body including:

- Cellular roles: Fats are integral to the structure of cell membranes.
- Protection and insulation: Fat layers cushion your organs and insulate you against the cold.
- Vitamin transport: Vitamins A, D, E and K are fat-soluble - meaning that they need fats for transport and absorption.
- Hormonal functions: Fats help to make vital hormones.

Not that fats are all created equal, and they are classified into several categories:

Saturated fats

These fats are typically solid at room temperature, and mainly found in animal sources like meat and dairy, and in some plant oils (like coconut oil). Their excessive consumption has been linked to heart disease, due to contributing towards cholesterol build-up (although it is important to note that research in to saturated fats in recent years has swung from them being "bad" to then having "no impact" – so the jury is still seems to be out on that one, and probably will be for many years).

Unsaturated fats

These heart-healthy fats are normally liquid at room temperature and fall in to two sub-groups:

- Monounsaturated fats (MUFAs): These are found in olive oil, avocados and many nuts. MUFAs are considered to be 'heart healthy'.
- Polyunsaturated fats (PUFAs): These are found in fish, flaxseeds and walnuts, and they include essential fatty acids like Omega-3 and Omega-6.

Trans fats

These are created from a process called hydrogenation (turning liquid fats into solids, primarily for shelf-life value) and are detrimental to health. While some trans fats occur naturally in meat and dairy, artificial trans fats (often found in processed foods) have been linked to increased heart disease risk.

When it comes to type 2 diabetes, fats behave differently than carbohydrates. Unsaturated fats can actually improve insulin sensitivity, which is important for controlling blood sugar levels.

On the other hand, excessive consumption of saturated and trans fats can reduce insulin sensitivity. As type 2 diabetes and obesity often go hand in hand, managing weight is important and fats (being calorie-dense) should be consumed mindfully.

Type 2 diabetes can increase the risk of cardiovascular problems and heart disease, and therefore prioritising heart-healthy fats (as well as limiting saturated and trans fats) can help to reduce this risk.

>> ACTION POINTS - PRIORITY 1 <<

Pair wisely: When consuming carbohydrate-rich foods, pair them with healthy fats to slow sugar absorption
When enjoying carbohydrate-rich foods, like a slice of whole grain bread, add a spread of avocado or a handful of nuts on the side. These healthy fats help slow the release of sugars into your bloodstream, offering a steadier energy release. This small change not only enhances the nutritional profile of your meal but also supports better blood sugar control.

Monitor trans fats: Limit the intake of industrially-produced foods that may contain trans fats

When shopping, make a habit of glancing at the ingredients list on packaged foods. Words like "hydrogenated" or "partially hydrogenated" oils are telltale signs of trans fats. Opting for whole foods or products with shorter, recognisable ingredient lists can be a great strategy.

>> ACTION POINTS - PRIORITY 2 <<

Educate yourself: Delve deeper into understanding the different types of fats and their sources

Familiarise yourself with the common food sources for each type. When shopping, make it a habit to read food labels, noting the types of fats listed. This knowledge not only empowers you to make informed choices but also aids in ensuring a well-rounded diet.

Embrace healthy oils: Incorporate a variety of oils in your cooking (ensuring a balance of beneficial fats)

Next time you are shopping, pick up oils like olive, avocado, or flaxseed, each with unique flavour profiles and health benefits. Rotate these oils in your daily cooking, whether it is a drizzle over salads or in your favourite stir-fry. By varying your choices, you are not just enhancing taste, but also ensuring a mix of beneficial fatty acids.

Carb Counting

Carbohydrate counting can be a useful tool in the prevention and reversing type 2 diabetes. "Counting" may conjure up thoughts of equations and spreadsheets, but please let me assure you it is much simpler and empowering than you might think.

Carbohydrate counting is about having a more detailed understanding of the food you consume. With that knowledge comes the power to make informed decisions, to enjoy a variety of foods and to maintain stable blood sugar levels.

Instead of avoiding certain foods altogether, carbohydrate counting gives you some freedom to make choices based on knowledge. For example, if you know how many carbohydrates are in a slice of whole grain bread or an apple, you can factor them into your daily intake, ensuring you neither deprive yourself nor overindulge.

The first step is to recognise sources of carbohydrates in your diet (we covered these earlier). Another useful skill is to read and understand food labels, and on packaged foods you will find a 'carbohydrates' section (which shows the total amount of carbohydrates per serving) - this is a key number to consider when carbohydrate counting.

The label will also break down carbohydrates into sugars and possibly fibre, giving you a clearer idea of what you are consuming. Besides the food label, there are several useful mobile phone apps where you can search for the carbohydrate content of various foods, including those that are rarely labelled, like fruits and vegetables.

While those numbers are helpful, it is essential to remember the quality of carbohydrates you are consuming. Remember, choosing whole and minimally processed foods provides you with complex carbohydrates and essential vitamins, minerals and fibre that support overall health.

As you grow more familiar with counting, you will find it easier to balance your daily intake. It is all about harmony and ensuring you provide your body with steady energy while managing blood sugar levels.

Begin by writing down what you eat and its carbohydrate count. Over time, doing this can offer you insights into dietary patterns – perhaps you notice that certain combinations keep you feeling fuller for longer or that certain foods cause a faster spike in blood sugar than you expected.

>> ACTION POINTS - PRIORITY 1 <<

Read labels: Limit your 'total' carbohydrate consumption to no more than 40g per meal
Whilst complex carbohydrates form part of a balanced diet, too many can be a problem. Using a food diary app, try to keep the maximum number of total (all) carbohydrates to no more than 40g per meal.

Read labels: Make a habit of checking food labels on packaged items, paying special attention to the carbohydrate section
Next time you are shopping, check the nutritional information on the packaging and look for the section that lists 'carbohydrates'. This figure is important and, over time, this quick check will become routine and will help you make better-informed choices.

Education: Spend time getting to know the carbohydrate content of the food you consume regularly
Begin by examining food labels when grocery shopping, noting their carbohydrate content. Initially, focus on familiarising yourself with the foods you eat most often and, as you get more comfortable, expand your knowledge to a broader range of foods.

Quality over quantity: Remember, it is not just about the numbers
While counting carbohydrates is useful, the quality of those carbohydrates matters immensely. Instead of reaching for processed foods that might fit your carbohydrate count, opt for whole foods like

vegetables, fruits, and whole grains. These not only provide essential nutrients, but also support stable blood sugar levels. Start by incorporating one or two whole foods into each meal, gradually increasing as you feel comfortable.

>> ACTION POINT - PRIORITY 2 <<

Journaling: For a week or two, keep a food diary and note down foods and their corresponding carbohydrate counts

Starting a food diary can be a game-changer in understanding how carbohydrates affect your blood sugar. Grab a notebook and jot down everything you eat, alongside its carbohydrate count. You can easily find these counts on food labels or one of the many apps as noted. For an added layer of insight, write down your blood sugar readings before and 2 hours after each meal. Over time, you will spot patterns, helping you make better-informed food choices.

Glycaemic Index and Glycaemic Load

Having a basic understanding of the glycaemic index and glycaemic load can be helpful in blood sugar control. In simple terms, glycaemic index and glycaemic load are ways to help you understand how different foods affect your blood sugar levels. You really do not need a deep understanding of this subject, but an overview of how it all works is useful.

The glycaemic index (GI) provides a measure of how quickly a carbohydrate-containing food raises blood glucose levels compared to pure glucose. Foods high on the GI scale raise blood sugar rapidly, whereas those lower on the scale provide a steadier energy release.

Glycaemic load (GL) considers both the quality and quantity of carbohydrates, and it gives a more comprehensive picture. By considering the GI and the volume of carbohydrates in a typical serving of food, it better reflects a food's real-life impact on blood sugar.

Consuming high GI foods regularly can cause rapid spikes in blood sugar, which forces your body to produce more insulin. Therefore, prioritising low and medium GI foods (as well as controlling portion sizes, and therefore the GL) can help maintain more stable blood sugar levels.

Low GI foods take longer to digest and absorb, helping you feel fuller for longer, which can help in weight management, too. Beyond just type 2 diabetes, a diet oriented towards low GI foods has been associated with reduced risks of heart disease, certain cancers, and other health issues.

Low GI (55 or less): Foods that release glucose slowly and steadily

Examples include:
- Most whole fruits (e.g. apples, pears, oranges, plums)
- Non-starchy vegetables
- Legumes (e.g. beans, lentils, chickpeas)
- Whole grain bread and cereals (e.g., barley, bran, oat bran)
- Pasta (al dente)
- Dairy products (e.g., milk, yogurt)
- Sweet potatoes
- Nuts and seeds

Medium GI (56-69): Foods that release glucose at a moderate rate

Examples include:
- Whole wheat, rye and pita bread
- Instant oats
- Brown, wild, or basmati rice
- Couscous
- Beetroots

- Pineapple
- Raisins

High GI (70 and above): Foods that release glucose quickly

Examples include:
- Rice cakes
- Most processed breakfast cereals
- Instant oatmeal
- Short-grain white rice
- Pretzels
- Saltine crackers
- Potatoes (boiled or mashed)
- Watermelon
- Dates

To calculate the glycaemic load of a food:

GL= (GI multiplied by the amount of carbohydrate per serving) ÷ 100

For practical purposes, GL can be categorised as:
- Low (10 or less): Indicates a minimal rise in blood sugar.
- Medium (11-19): Signifies a moderate impact on blood sugar.
- High (20 or more): Suggests a high impact on blood sugar.

The glycaemic load in action:

Watermelon:
- GI: High (72).
- However, a small serving (100g) of watermelon does not have a lot of carbohydrates (7g).
- (72 x 7) ÷ 100 = a GL of 5, placing it in the low GL category.

2 slices of white bread:
- GI: High (around 75).
- A typical slice (29g) has about 15g of carbohydrates.
- (75 x 30) ÷ 100 = a GL of 22.5, placing it in the high GL category.

Red lentil pasta (cooked al dente):
- GI: Low (around 22).
- A 100g serving has 61g of carbohydrates.
- (22 x 61) ÷ 100 = a GL of 13, placing it in the medium category.

White pasta (cooked al dente):
- GI: Low (around 55).
- A 100g serving has 70g of carbohydrates.
- (55 x 70) ÷ 100 = a GL of 38, placing it in the high category.

Red split lentils:

- GI: Low (around 21).
- A serving might contain around 40g of carbohydrates.
- (21 x 40) ÷ 100 = a GL of 8.4, placing it in the low GL category.

>> ACTION POINTS - PRIORITY 1 <<

Balance your meals: Combining different foods can influence the overall glycaemic index of a meal

When preparing your meals, keep balance in mind. If you are planning a dish that is rich in higher glycaemic index carbohydrates, like rice, consider adding a protein source like grilled chicken or a healthy fat such as avocado. This does not just enhance flavour, but can help moderate the blood sugar response, making your meal more blood sugar friendly. Over time, you will get a feel for combinations that work best for you, promoting steady energy and steady blood sugars.

Consider the overall balance of your meals, incorporating proteins and fats to manage the glycaemic impact

Achieving a well-balanced meal is like crafting a harmonious melody, that is you do not want one instrument overpowering the others. Similarly, blend carbohydrates with vegetables, sources of protein like lean meats, fish or beans and healthy fats such as avocados or nuts. This mix not only makes meals more satisfying but also helps smooth out rapid spikes in blood sugar.

Whole foods first: Natural, minimally processed foods often have a more favourable glycaemic index profile

Vegetables (except for potatoes and many other root vegetables), fruits, whole grains and lean proteins usually have a more stable effect on blood sugar. When shopping, prioritise items that resemble their natural state and avoid those with flashy packaging or extensive ingredient lists. Not only will you be choosing foods with a better glycaemic profile, but you will also nourish your body with essential nutrients.

>> ACTION POINT - PRIORITY 2 <<

Be mindful, not obsessive: Use glycaemic index and glycaemic load as tools, not strict rules

While the glycaemic index and glycaemic load offer valuable insights into how the foods you eat impact your blood sugar, they are simply guidance. Rather than rigidly sticking to low glycaemic index foods alone, embrace a varied diet. Let the glycaemic index and glycaemic load be gentle reminders, not regimented rules. Balance is key and joy in eating is essential too.

Fibre

Dietary fibre is an important part of blood sugar control, and one that is often not well understood or is simply overlooked. Consuming an adequate amount of daily fibre has several health benefits, not least of which is to contribute to stable blood sugar levels.

Fibre is the indigestible parts of plant-based foods we eat. Unlike carbohydrates, proteins and fats, our body cannot break down fibre and digest it. Instead, it travels through the digestive tract - and during that journey through the body, it plays a key role in our health.

There are two main types of fibre: soluble and insoluble - each has its unique set of benefits.

Soluble fibre
Derived from the Latin word 'solubilis' meaning 'soluble,' this type of fibre dissolves in water, forming a gel-like consistency in the gut, and slowing down the digestion process and the absorption rate of sugar in the bloodstream. This means that after a meal, blood sugar levels rise at a more gradual pace, preventing abrupt spikes. Because of its nature, soluble fibre also adds bulkiness to meals, instilling a sense of fullness. This not only helps you to feel satiated for longer but also can aid in weight management.

Beyond its effects on glucose, soluble fibre helps reduce the levels of LDL cholesterol and this is important for type 2 diabetics, as they often have an elevated risk of heart-related conditions. Soluble fibre is great for gut health too, helping to feed and maintain your symbiotic relationship with your 100 trillion (or so) gut bacteria. The more you feed them and keep them healthy, the more they reciprocate and help you with your health.

Sources of soluble fibre

- Unprocessed oats: A staple breakfast option, and steel cuts oats in particular can be a good way to increase soluble fibre intake.
- Beans and lentils: Besides being protein rich, these are excellent sources of soluble fibre.
- Fruits: Apples, pears and citrus fruits are great forms of soluble fibre.
- Vegetables: Most vegetables contain high levels of soluble fibre.
- Seeds and husks: Chia seeds and psyllium husks are an excellent source of soluble fibre.

Insoluble fibre

Insoluble fibre does not dissolve in water and its primary role is to add bulk to faecal matter, which aids efficient digestion. By adding bulk to stools, insoluble fibre ensures smooth bowel movements, preventing conditions like constipation. In relation to type 2 diabetes, and through encouraging a consistent digestive process, insoluble fibre also plays an indirect role in helping to maintain steady blood sugar levels.

Sources of insoluble fibre:

- Whole grains: Foods like whole grain bread, brown rice and barley are good sources of insoluble fibre.
- Vegetables: Green beans, cauliflower and sweet potatoes are great sources of insoluble fibre.
- Nuts and seeds: Not only are they a good source of insoluble fibre, but are good for increasing protein intake too.

>> ACTION POINTS - PRIORITY 1 <<

Fibre tracking: For a few days, track your daily fibre intake
*Keep a diary of everything you eat and jot down the fibre content (easily found on food labels or quick online searches). After a few days, add up your daily averages. If you are falling short of the **25-30g** daily target, then perhaps it is time for a tweak. Maybe introduce a handful of berries at breakfast, include a piece of fruit (with its peel) as a daily snack or add a tablespoon of chia seed to your Greek yoghurt. If your current diet is low in fibre, then build on it gradually, working towards the daily target over a month. Small, conscious changes can make a big difference.*

Natural over processed: Try to incorporate one additional natural fibre source into your meals daily
Start with small changes: the next time you make a salad, toss in a handful of kidney beans or chickpeas. Fancy a snack? Reach for an apple or a pear with its peel. And when you are at the shop, choose red

lentil or pea pasta over its white counterpart. These tiny shifts will not only add delicious textures and flavours, but will also help ensure a healthier fibre intake, supporting better blood sugar control and overall wellbeing.

>> ACTION POINT - PRIORITY 2 <<

Audit your food cupboard: Over the next week, review the fibre content of foods in your food cupboard

Over the coming week, set aside some time to examine the labels on your food items, focusing on their fibre content. It might surprise you at what is lurking in so-called healthy products. If a particular food is lacking in fibre, jot it down. Next time you are shopping, seek fibre-rich alternatives.

Omega-3 and Omega-6

You may have heard of 'Omega-3' and 'Omega-6' fats, and you might know that Omega-3 is commonly found in fish. Beyond that, few people understand what these essential fatty acids are, what they do and why balancing them against each other is important for good health.

Omega-3 (O3) and Omega-6 (O6) are both polyunsaturated fats (the healthy fats as we learnt about earlier), and they are termed 'essential' because your body cannot produce them - and you need to get them from your diet.

O3 fatty acids are recognised for being good for the heart and cardiovascular system, as they can help decrease inflammation, reduce the risk of heart disease and even support brain function. You can get O3 from fish, especially oily types like salmon and mackerel, or from non-fish sources like flaxseeds, chia seeds, and walnuts.

O6 fatty acids come primarily from plant oils, including sunflower, corn and soybean. While they have their place in a balanced diet and can be beneficial for brain function and supporting growth and development, an over-consumption of O6 can lead to health problems including water retention, high blood pressure and chronic inflammation (chronic inflammation can be the precursor to insulin resistance).

Our ancestors probably consumed O3 and O6 in a balanced ratio since they had fewer O6-rich foods in their diet compared to us today. Our modern diet has seen a surge in O6 consumption, which has upset the 3-to-6 balance. Processed foods, which often contain plant-based oils, have led to a significant increase in our intake of O6 instead of O3.

Do not try to eliminate O6 altogether (as that would create other issues including dry skin, brittle nails, increased risk of infection and poor wound healing), instead be aware of it in your diet and ensure you are not overindulging. Simple steps like checking the ingredients list of processed foods, snacks and salad dressings can help to reduce your O6 intake and cooking with olive or avocado oil (which have a more balanced O3 to O6 ratio) rather than plant-based oils can help too.

Striking the right balance between O3 and O6 is about making conscious choices, understanding the sources, and consciously moving the balance towards a more natural consumption pattern. Regularly consuming O3 rich foods and being cautious of excessive O6's can help to improve your health.

>> ACTION POINTS - PRIORITY 1 <<

Assess your diet: Reflect on your current Omega-3 intake and identify areas for enhancement
Start by jotting down the foods you typically eat in a week. Once you have a list, look specifically for sources of Omega-3 like fish, walnuts and flaxseeds. If these foods appear infrequently or not at all, it is a nudge to incorporate more of them into your meals.

Limit the consumption of processed foods and check labels to understand Omega-6 content
Cutting back on processed foods is a positive step towards balancing your Omega intake. Many of these foods sneakily have high Omega-6 levels, often from refined oils. Begin by looking at the ingredients list and if you spot oils (like vegetable, sunflower, soybean, or corn oil) it is a hint about its Omega-6 content.

Maintain balance: Be mindful of your Omega-6 intake, striving to maintain a balanced ratio with Omega-3s
Achieving a balanced intake of Omega-3 and Omega-6 is vital for optimal health. Start by being conscious of foods rich in Omega-6. Instead, lean towards foods abundant in Omega-3. Regularly reviewing food labels can help you monitor your intake. Over time, this mindful eating will naturally guide you towards a balanced Omega ratio.

Choose healthier cooking oils, like olive or avocado oil, for a balanced fatty acid intake

Next time you are shopping, take a moment to explore the oil section. Look for olive or avocado oil as these oils not only impart a pleasant flavour but also offer a better balance of fatty acids compared to many other cooking oils.

>> ACTION POINTS - PRIORITY 2 <<

Diversify sources: Introduce a mix of both animal and plant-based sources of Omega-3s to your diet

For a well-rounded Omega-3 intake, it is good to embrace variety. You might enjoy salmon or mackerel one day and then switch to plant-based sources like chia seeds or walnuts the next. This not only ensures you are getting different types of Omega-3's, but also adds a mix of textures and flavours to your meals.

Seek quality: Opt for high-quality sources of these fats, such as wild-caught fish or organic seeds

When selecting your Omega-rich foods, quality truly counts. Instead of just any fish, choose wild-caught options (which often have a purer Omega-3 content). To avoid unwanted chemicals, select organic flax or chia seeds when buying.

Fruit

One of the most popular topics raised by my clients is that of fruit, and specifically of fruit's impact on blood sugars. Some sources say that fruit should be avoided altogether, whilst others say that fruit is okay in moderation. I fall into the latter category, as the health benefits of eating fruit far outweigh any issues that might be caused by the naturally occurring sugars.

In their natural and unprocessed form, fruit has a range of beneficial nutrients and a bounty of fibre (especially in their skins). This fibre slows down the absorption of sugar during digestion, and helping to stabilise blood sugar levels, as we learnt in the previous section.

However, not all fruits are created equal when it comes to how their sugars affect your blood sugars and, whilst there are many fruits to enjoy (in moderation), there are some that you would do well to steer clear of (including fruit derivatives).

Here are some examples.

Fruits that have a lesser impact on blood sugars (can be enjoyed in moderation)
- Apples (preferably with skin)
- Pears (preferably with skin)

- Cherries
- Grapefruit
- Oranges
- Plums
- Strawberries
- Kiwifruit
- Blueberries
- Blackberries
- Raspberries
- Guava
- Avocado
- Passionfruit
- Limes
- Nectarines
- Peaches
- Apricots
- Figs (fresh)

Fruits that might cause problems with blood sugar levels (better to avoid or consume less often / in smaller quantities)

- Watermelon
- Pineapple
- Ripe bananas
- Lychee
- Dates
- Raisins

- Currants
- Prunes
- Mangos (especially when ripe)
- Papaya
- Overripe kiwi
- Overripe peaches
- Fruit cocktail blends with added sugars
- Dried fruits coated with added sugar
- Canned fruits in syrup
- Grapes (can be higher GI than other fruits)
- Persimmons
- Fruit juices (even 100% fruit juice can spike blood sugar rapidly)
- Fruit smoothies, especially those with added sugars or honey

Fruit has its place in your diet - but is all about making informed choices, understanding the effects on your own blood sugar and enjoying them as part of a balanced diet. While they contain naturally occurring sugars, when chosen wisely, consumed in the right portions and eaten as part of a balanced diet, fruit is without doubt beneficial. You might find is a useful exercise to check your blood sugar levels 30 minutes after eating any fruit, as this will give you a good idea of its impact on your body.

>> ACTION POINTS - PRIORITY 1 <<

Opt for whole: Choose fresh or frozen whole fruits over fruit juices or dried fruits

Next time you shop, pick up some fresh apples, berries, or oranges instead of reaching for fruit juice or dried fruits. Whole fruits offer the satisfaction of natural sweetness, combined with beneficial fibre that helps steady sugar absorption. But remember, even with fruit, the poison is in the dose, so enjoy them, but choose carefully and eat in moderation.

Be conscious of portions: Keep an eye on portion sizes

Being mindful of portion sizes with fruit can make a difference in blood sugar control. Instead of guessing, simply visualise: think of a handful when you opt for berries, choose a fruit that fits comfortably in your palm.

>> ACTION POINT - PRIORITY 2 <<

Mind the pairing: The next time you enjoy fruit, pair it with a protein or healthy fat source

Pairing fruits with a protein or healthy fat can slow down the release of sugars, giving you sustained energy. Why not spread a little almond or peanut butter on your apple slices, or perhaps spoon some creamy Greek yoghurt over your fresh berries?

Fructose

Fructose is the naturally occurring sugar found in fruit, honey and some vegetables (asparagus, cauliflower, green peppers, leafy greens, celery, mushrooms, cucumber, and root vegetables). However, the fructose found naturally in whole fruits (and vegetables) is not the same as the extracted fructose that can be found in some processed and almost all ultra-processed foods.

Alongside the fructose consumed when you eat a piece of fruit, you are also taking in fibre, vitamins and other nutrients. The fibre in fruit helps regulate your blood sugar by slowing down the release of natural sugars into your bloodstream.

However, the story changes **SIGNIFICANTLY** when fructose is taken from its natural environment and served on its own either as fruit juices or added to foods and drinks.

In many manufactured foods and drinks, fructose has been extracted from natural sources and then processed to create high fructose corn syrup (HFCS). HFCS is cheaper, sweeter and more flexible in its use than normal white table sugar, which makes it a go-to choice for food companies. However, unlike the natural fructose found in fruit, HFCS does not come with the good stuff - the beneficial fibre and nutrients. As a result, this extracted fructose is absorbed much more rapidly, leading to quicker and higher spikes in blood sugar levels.

The damage caused by this HFCS goes beyond our blood sugars. Because it is the liver that processes fructose, when you consume it in large amounts, your liver can become overloaded. It then converts the excess fructose into fat and, over time, this can contribute to problems like non-alcoholic fatty liver disease (NAFLD) which can affect your blood sugar levels and insulin sensitivity.

Another consideration regarding the over consumption of fructose from processed/ultra-processed foods is its inability to satisfy us. This means you might end up consuming more calories than you realise, which over time can lead to weight gain and other health issues.

What if you are trying to control your blood sugars?

It is important to remember that not all fructose sources are equal, and the fructose found in whole fruits (when consumed in moderation) can contribute to a balanced diet as they offer vitamins, antioxidants and essential fibre. The problems come from 'extracted' fructose, that is, fructose that is consumed away from its natural source. I encourage you to check the food labels of any manufactured foods and drinks you might buy, and look for ingredients like "high fructose corn syrup" or "fructose syrup." These are clear signs that the product contains this extracted and dangerous form of fructose.

Do not fear fructose - but understand where it comes from in your food and consume it in moderation (and then only from natural sources).

>> ACTION POINTS - PRIORITY 1 <<

Embrace whole fruits: Enjoy fruits in their whole form
Choose whole fruits over fruit-based products. The next time you fancy a sweet treat, reach for an apple or a handful of berries (instead of fruit juices or processed, sugary snacks).

Read labels: Next time you are shopping, check the labels
When you are out shopping, look at ingredient lists. Keep an eye out for "high fructose corn syrup", "fructose syrup" or "glucose syrup". Recognising these names will help you make informed choices and will help you avoid unnecessary added sugars in your diet. Make a point of completely avoiding foods where you see "fructose" of any kind in the ingredients list on processed foods or drinks.

Limit sugary drinks: Reduce or eliminate fizzy drinks and overly sweet drinks from your diet.
Reducing your sugary drink intake can make a significant difference in your fructose consumption. If you enjoy fizzy, sugary drinks, start by swapping one or two cans a day for a couple of glasses of water (carbonated or non-carbonated) or a herbal/green tea. Then gradually wean yourself off of them completely. When out and about, choose your drinks wisely - take a moment to read the ingredients list on the label,

keeping an eye out for high fructose corn syrup or artificial sweeteners.

Cakes, Biscuits, Drinks and Sweets

Given that one of the primary drivers of high blood sugar is simple, refined and processed sugars, I could summarise this section by simply advising you to avoid sugary sweets, drinks, cakes, biscuits and snacks altogether - and to be fair, that would be good advice.

However, it would be good to briefly review the reasons I suggest you abstain from these foods and drinks (or certainly consume them in minimal quantities).

Sugary foods and drinks not only cause a quick surge in blood sugar levels, but are also mostly empty calories and devoid of essential nutrients. Over consumption of these can lead to weight gain, which then can complicate blood sugar management further. Sugar, whether in its obvious forms like table sugar or hidden in processed foods under pseudonyms like high-fructose corn syrup, is associated with other health issues ranging from heart disease to the development of certain cancers.

To tackle the sugar monster, it is important to be equipped with strategies that support you in making healthier choices without imposing a feeling of deprivation. Staying hydrated is essential as often the body misinterprets thirst as hunger, which can then lead you to reach for a sugary treat when a simple glass of water could suffice.

If you feel that you are on the sugar-addiction roller-coaster, then take time to review 'breaking the sugar addiction cycle' covered earlier.

Natural sweeteners and fruit can provide sweetness, but without the negative effects of processed sugars. Ensure your diet comprises a balance of proteins, fats, and complex carbohydrates - as these can help you control your blood sugar levels and curb those sugar cravings.

>> ACTION POINTS - PRIORITY 1 <<

Cut them out: To conquer type 2 diabetes, these must be kept to an absolute minimum (ideally, cut out altogether)
There is no easy way to say this, but cakes, biscuits, sweets, chocolate, sugary drinks... these will all drive your blood sugars up, and quickly. Breaking away from them is easier said than done, I know, but is essential. If you consume a lot of these types of products, initially try to wean yourself off them, bit by bit, day by day. Consciously try to eat less and you will find that the cravings subside over time - but it takes conscious effort to break free (refer to the 'Sugar Addiction Cycle' and How We Create Habits' sections).

Find suitable replacements (like fruit, for example) and do your best to keep away from the foods/drinks you are tempted by (for example, do not have them in your home – if you do not have easy access to them, the chances are that cravings will quickly pass, and you will naturally consume less).

Hydration challenge: Aim to replace at least one sugary drink a day with water or an unsweetened alternative

The next time you are about to reach for a fizzy drink or fruit juice, pause. Instead, opt for a glass of water or perhaps a herbal tea without added sugars. If you miss the fizz, then sparkling water can be a suitable replacement. Making this switch helps cut sugar and keeps you well-hydrated. Over time, you might even prefer these to sugary alternatives.

Label detective: Make it a habit to check the sugar content on food labels

Next time you are shopping, find the "carbohydrates of which sugars" section on the nutritional label. Compare products and select ones with lower sugar. Over time, this habit will help you make better choices.

Audit your food cupboard: Take a look at what is in your kitchen

Go through your food cupboard and take out products and check their labels for sugar content, (especially those items you consume often). Surprised by what you find? That is to be expected and is okay. Replace sugary food and snacks with healthier options.

Healthy Snacking

When 'snacks' are mentioned, many people likely imagine bags of crisps, sugary biscuits, or chocolate bars. These processed snacks are high in sugar, fat, and calories, and simply will not help you prevent or reverse type 2 diabetes. On the other hand, healthy snacks can bridge the gap between meals, can offer an additional source of essential nutrients and will often have little impact on blood sugar levels.

A 'healthy' snack should be as natural as possible (be actual food and not some manufactured facsimile), be nutritionally balanced and provide a mix of protein, healthy fats, and some complex carbohydrates. This combination ensures a steady release of energy.

Some healthy snack ideas
- Nuts and seeds: A small handful of almonds, walnuts, or pumpkin seeds can be a powerhouse of nutrition - providing protein, healthy fats, and some carbohydrates.
- Yoghurt with berries: Choose natural or Greek yoghurt, topped with a mix of berries. This snack offers a good balance of protein, carbohydrates and antioxidants.

- Hummus and veggie sticks: Hummus, made from chickpeas, provides protein and healthy fats. Paired with vegetables like cucumber or carrot sticks, it becomes a nutritious snack.
- Boiled eggs: Easily portable, boiled eggs are a source of high-quality protein and essential vitamins.
- Whole grain crackers with avocado: A slice of avocado on a whole grain cracker can offer healthy fats, fibre, as well as essential vitamins and minerals.

>> ACTION POINTS - PRIORITY 1 <<

Stay hydrated: Sometimes we confuse thirst with hunger
Often, your body might signal hunger when you are actually thirsty. Before reaching for a snack, drink a medium to large glass of water and then give it a few minutes. You might find that the water quenches your thirst and what were perceived as hunger pangs subside. This simple habit can help ensure you are eating in response to genuine hunger, rather than a misinterpreted thirst signal.

Read labels: If opting for packaged snacks, scrutinise the label
When choosing packaged snacks, always be on the lookout! Turn that packet around and look at the label. Check for any added sugars, making sure they are not sneaking into your snack. Also, look at the balance of protein, fats and carbohydrates. Choose snacks that offer a mix of these macronutrients. By making label-reading a regular habit, you will empower yourself to make informed snacking choices.

Assess your snacking habits: Are your current snacks aiding or hindering your health goals?

Write down the snacks you eat in a week. Then, assess each snack for protein, healthy fats, and complex carbohydrates. Are they free from excessive sugars and unhealthy additives? If you find that many of your snacks do not align with your health goals, it is a gentle nudge to reconsider (and swap them out for more nutritious options).

Stay mindful: Approach snacking with mindfulness, focusing on both quality and quantity

Mindful snacking is about fully engaging in the moment, savouring each bite and recognising your body's hunger and fullness signals. Start by choosing nutrient-rich snacks, then set them on a plate rather than eating from a packet. Find a quiet spot, away from distractions. As you eat, focus on the texture, flavour and how the snack makes you feel. By giving your full attention to what you are consuming and how much, you will probably find yourself more satisfied.

Getting your snack portions right can make a world of difference, so begin by familiarising yourself with the recommended serving sizes, which can often be found on packaging. Then, instead of snacking directly from a packet, measure out the correct portion onto a plate or bowl. Over time, this simple habit can help train your eye to recognise appropriate amounts. Remember, it is not just about what you eat that matters, but also how much.

>> ACTION POINTS - PRIORITY 2 <<

Plan ahead: Stock up on healthy snack options (so you are not tempted by less nutritious alternatives)

Before your next shopping trip, make a list of healthy snacks, such as nuts, seeds or Greek yoghurt. When you are at the shop, stick to your list, resisting the temptation of sugary or processed snacks. Once home, allocate a dedicated 'healthy snack' shelf or drawer, making it easier to grab a nutritious snack when hunger strikes. By having these better-for-you snacks readily accessible, you will be naturally steering your snacking habits towards making better choices.

Monitor blood sugar levels: As you incorporate healthy snacks, keep track of your blood sugar levels to understand how different foods impact them

As you introduce healthier snacks into your diet, use a home blood sugar testing kit at regular intervals, noting down the readings alongside what you have eaten. Over time, this will give you a good idea of how specific snacks influence your levels. Remember, consistency is key – test around the same times each day for accurate comparisons. This practice will not only empower you with knowledge but also guide you in fine-tuning your snack choices.

Processed and Ultra Processed Foods

Despite knowing the advantages of whole foods, why do people opt for other options or not consume them regularly?

The reason is simple - we live in an age of convenience where unhealthy food is readily available in supermarkets, and their shelves are packed with ready-made meals, canned foods, and high-calorie low-nutrient snacks in eye-catching packaging. And that is before we even take in to account the growth of fast-food outlets in many countries.

Yes, the temptation of processed and ultra-processed foods is all around us, and there is nothing quite like added salt, sugar or fat to get you hooked on to them (and the food manufacturers are masters in knowing how to make their processed foods additive).

However, if you are looking to improve your health, then you really need to be aware of the problems associated with some processed foods - and try to avoid ultra-processed foods altogether. Let us now distinguish the two types.

A 'processed' food is one that has been altered from its natural state, sometimes for safety reasons, often for convenience and frequently for taste. This means not all processed foods are inherently bad as, for instance, pasteurised milk is processed, but it is done to eliminate harmful bacteria.

'Ultra-processed' foods go much further than processed foods and are products that have undergone multiple processes, and have many (normally ten or more) added ingredients (such as sugar, unhealthy trans fats and artificial additives). They bear little or no resemblance to real food and the giveaway is their long ingredients list - often filled with substances not typically used in home cooking, and many of which cannot even be pronounced!

Some processed foods - and especially ultra-processed foods - come laden with 'extras' that are not good for your health, including colourings, flavour enhancers, emulsifiers, added sugar, added unhealthy fats, and added salt. On top of that, they often offer little in terms of the things that are good for you - like vitamins, minerals and other essential nutrients.

As these foods are generally calorie-dense and nutrient sparse, the frequent consumption of these foods can significantly increase your caloric intake and also leave you feeling unsatisfied - which then leads in to overeating and so the cycle continues. Over time, this can cause weight gain, which is a big risk factor with type 2 diabetes.

Many processed and ultra-processed foods, even those not necessarily sweet, can contain added sugars and trans-fats - both of which have been linked to increased heart disease risk. There is often a high salt content in these types of food too, and a high sodium intake is associated with elevated blood pressure.

Let me leave you with a concluding thought on ultra-processed food... just because something is edible does **NOT** make it 'food'!

>> ACTION POINTS - PRIORITY 1 <<

Audit your food cupboard: Check your current food items
Begin by emptying one shelf at a time and categorising each item: natural, lightly processed, or ultra processed. For those that fall into the last category, jot down possible healthier swaps. Maybe switch that sugary cereal for steel-cut oats or crisps for unsalted nuts. By actively recognising and replacing, you are setting yourself up for better choices on your next shop.

Read labels: Look for products with minimal added sugars, salts, and unhealthy fats
Look at the ingredient list of products. Keep an eye out for ingredients like sucrose, fructose, high fructose corn syrup, corn syrup and glucose syrup – these are just different names for sugar. Products with fewer added sugars, salts and unhealthy fats are better choices. Over time, recognising these names and opting for simpler ingredient lists will

become second nature, helping you make healthier, informed decisions.

Check ingredients: A shorter ingredient list often indicates a less processed product
As a rule, shorter lists often point towards less processed foods. If you can recognise and pronounce most of the ingredients, that is usually a good sign. Over time, this quick scan will become a habit, guiding you towards informed choices.

>> ACTION POINTS - PRIORITY 2 <<

Plan meals in advance: By planning, you are less likely to choose convenience foods
Start by jotting down a menu for the upcoming days, keeping in mind the balance of nutrients you would like to achieve. Once you have a plan, create a shopping list filled with fresh, whole ingredients. This not only ensures you have everything you need at hand, but also reduces those last-minute temptations to reach for a processed convenience option. Over time, this simple habit will make it second nature to choose nourishing meals that support your health and wellbeing.

Cook at home: Try new recipes and explore home-cooked meals
Begin with simple recipes that feature whole foods you love and, over time, experiment with different herbs, spices, and fresh produce. Cooking at home not only lets you select high-quality ingredients but also helps with portion control.

Whole Foods

Whole foods are foods in their natural and unaltered state (or with minimal processing). Think of carrots pulled fresh from the earth, apples plucked from a tree, or grains harvested from the fields. These foods are natural, are packed with nourishment, and are essential for good health - as they typically contain a range of vitamins, minerals, fibre and antioxidants. With no need for preservation, colouring, or artificial flavourings, whole foods are free from many chemicals and additives that processed foods often contain, and their fibre content helps with digestion, enhances satiety and plays a key role in blood sugar regulation.

The relationship between whole foods and blood sugar control is intertwined. Due to their high fibre content, whole foods tend to release glucose into the bloodstream slowly, which helps to reduce blood sugar spikes. Whole foods can naturally help your body to improve its insulin response too, as nutrients like magnesium (present in whole grains and green leafy vegetables), have been shown to improve insulin sensitivity. In addition to the vitamins, minerals and fibre found in whole foods, they are also high in antioxidants and other protective compounds, and these can help reduce the risk of common diabetic complications, including heart disease and neuropathy.

Whole foods can also be great in helping with weight management/loss too, as they are "nutrient-dense and calorie-sparse" (unlike most processed food that is nutrient-sparse and calorie-dense, dwell on that concept for a moment…), and so because you chew whole foods more, you will naturally eat less.

It is worthy of note that whilst whole foods will always be better for your health than processed or ultra-processed foods, some vegetables (particularly starchy and below-the-ground (root) vegetables can cause blood sugar spikes. Of note are potatoes in any form. From my experience, potatoes cause quick and significant increases in blood sugar levels every time, regardless of how they are presented (boiled, mashed, chipped etc…). If you want to find out how specific vegetables affect your blood sugars, using a CGM or fingerprick glucose monitor alongside a food diary for a month will give you a clearer picture.

The contrast between processed foods and whole foods could not be more striking. Processed (and highly/ultra processed) foods often strip away essential nutrients during their production (yes, they often take out the healthy stuff in food that makes it good for you!). What you are left with is high sugar/fat/salt real food facsimiles that are a poor excuse for 'food'. These can raise blood sugar levels, hamper insulin sensitivity and, over time, cause a raft of other health problems from heart disease to cancer.

>> ACTION POINTS - PRIORITY 1 <<

Make wise choices: Choose whole foods whenever you can
You cannot beat the power of whole, natural foods in providing you with the nourishment that you need to survive and thrive. Situations may arise when you have no choice but to consume food from a packet or tin, but where possible, make a concerted effort to choose food in its natural, unprocessed form. Do remember, however, that you can have too much of a good thing, and portion size is important. In addition, remember that 'below the ground' (root) vegetables cause more pronounced blood sugar spikes than does above the ground veg.

Stay committed: Remember, every meal is an opportunity to nourish your body
Each time you are about to eat, pause for a moment. Take a few seconds to reflect on the commitment you have made to improve your health. Ask yourself if what you are about to eat will take you slightly closer to your goal, or further from it. This act of pausing can break the automatic process of eating, and can steer you towards more nutritious and healthier options - and away from fleeting temptations.

>> ACTION POINTS - PRIORITY 2 <<

Audit your food cupboard: Look at what is in your kitchen
Start by setting aside a little time to go through your food cupboard and

identify those items which are heavily processed or high in added sugars. On your next shopping trip, seek whole food replacements for these unhealthy foods. For instance, swap sugary cereals with steel-cut oats or processed snacks with nuts, seeds or fruit.

Document your journey: Keep a journal of your move to a more whole foods-based diet - noting any changes in your energy, mood and blood sugar levels

Set aside a few moments each day to jot down your meals, how you felt, and any noticeable shifts in your energy and mood. Note any variations in your blood sugar readings if you monitor them. Over time, you will have a clear idea of the positive impact of whole foods are having on your health. This record not only serves as a motivational tool but also aids in fine-tuning your food choices.

Whole Grains

'Whole grains' are grains in their most natural form and encompass the entire seed of the plant. This includes the bran (the outer layer packed with fibre), the germ (the nutrient-rich core) and the endosperm (the middle layer containing starch). In contrast, bran and germ have been removed from refined grains, leaving only the starchy endosperm (which raises blood sugar levels quickly).

Distinguishing genuine whole grain products from non-whole varieties is a key step towards better blood sugar control. Reviewing ingredient lists for terms like 'whole' or 'whole grain' can be a good starting point.

Simple dietary switches, such as choosing brown rice over white rice or whole grain bread rather than white bread, can improve blood sugar control - and there is a fair range to choose from, including quinoa, oats and barley.

Whole grains are considerably richer in fibre compared to refined grains and, as we have learnt, fibre plays an important role in stabilising blood sugar levels by slowing the absorption of glucose into the bloodstream, as well as nurturing the gut's good bacteria and keeping them healthy too.

Look for words like 'whole' or 'whole grain' at the beginning of the ingredient list. Be wary of terms like 'multigrain' or '100% wheat', as they can be misleading and may not mean the product is made from whole grains.

A word of caution: whilst whole grains are infinitely better for you than refined and processed grains, even whole grains can raise blood sugar levels if eaten to excess. The key with grains is to minimise them, and then to only eat unprocessed whole grains products in moderation.

>> ACTION POINT - PRIORITY 1 <<

Read labels: When shopping, be vigilant
Keep an eye out for terms like 'whole' or 'whole grain' listed at the start, indicative of genuine whole grain content. For instance, 'whole wheat' or 'brown rice' are good signs, while terms like 'multigrain' might not guarantee whole grain benefits. Remember that even whole grains can raise blood sugar levels when consumed regularly or to excess, so moderation is important.

>> ACTION POINTS - PRIORITY 2 <<

Educate yourself: Get to know the variety of whole grains available (and their benefits)

Start by visiting your local supermarket's grain section, where you will probably find a variety of grains, from quinoa and oats to barley and millet. Take a moment to read the labels, noting their nutritional content.

Experiment in the kitchen: Try new recipes that incorporate whole grains

Begin by swapping out refined grains in your favourite recipes for their whole grain counterparts. Fancy a stir-fry? Use brown rice instead of white. Baking a loaf? Opt for whole grain flour. Explore online recipes that spotlight grains like quinoa in salads or barley in soups.

Hydration

Every system in your body relies on water - from the maintenance of body temperature to saliva production, from cardiovascular health to the final stages of digestion. Your kidneys rely heavily on adequate hydration to function properly too, and water also acts as a lubricant for your joints.

So, if you are dehydrated and not drinking enough water, how are your blood glucose levels affected?

Dehydration concentrates your blood, which leads to increased blood sugar levels as well as increased blood pressure. This increased blood sugar can then result in frequent urination, which can cause further dehydration. Drinking enough water each day helps your body function properly, including the insulin-producing cells in your pancreas. Type 2 diabetes can also place a strain on the kidneys, and ensuring proper hydration will help your kidneys to expel toxins which can reduce the risk of kidney issues.

Understanding the signs of dehydration is crucial, however for someone with type 2 diabetes these signs can sometimes be more pronounced:

- Frequent urination can be a symptom of high blood sugar levels, which can lead to dehydration.
- Persistent dry mouth and thirst is a common symptom, and also linked to frequent urination.
- Skin may appear dry and lack its usual elasticity.
- Feeling continually tired and fatigued can be an indicator of dehydration.
- As the brain relies heavily on water, dehydration can lead to headaches.

Proper hydration is an essential tool in blood sugar control. Other than drinking water, we can also hydrate ourselves by eating water-rich foods like fruits and vegetables, and drinking herbal/fruit/green teas. Remember to be careful with drinks such as alcohol, sugary drinks, and coffee as they can dehydrate you or affect blood sugar levels.

You cannot beat plain water for rehydrating yourself, but herbal teas can be a nice, caffeine-free alternative too. Milk provides essential nutrients (though it is best to choose unsweetened and unflavoured versions). On the other hand, fizzy drinks (which are often filled with sugars) can cause rapid blood sugar spikes, and even natural fruit juices - despite being perceived as healthy - can have high sugar levels and should be avoided. While a moderate amount of caffeine can be beneficial, consuming too much can cause dehydration and sleep disturbances.

Strategies to Stay Hydrated

- Start your day with water: Take a 250-500ml glass of water to bed with you and get in the habit of drinking it first thing in the morning upon waking.
- Set daily goals: Determine an optimal daily water intake and stick to it. A common recommendation is 8x8: eight 8-ounce (approx 250ml) glasses per day, but this varies based on individual needs.
- Use technology: There are many apps and smart bottles that help to remind you to drink water.
- Flavour your water: Add slices of cucumber, lemon, or fresh herbs to make water tastier.
- Hydrate throughout the day: Avoid consuming large amounts in one go - sip smaller amounts consistently instead.
- Monitor your urine colour: Aim for a pale straw colour as a sign of proper hydration.

>> ACTION POINTS - PRIORITY 1 <<

Track your intake: Document daily water consumption to ensure you are meeting your hydration target

Start by setting a daily water goal, like 2 or 2.5 litres, which can include non-caffeinated drinks and herbal teas. Then, simply make a note on your phone or in a diary each time you have a drink. There are also plenty of user-friendly apps available that can help you track and remind you to sip throughout the day.

Incorporate hydrating foods: Add water-rich foods to your meals and snacks

Hydration is not just about drinking water; it is about eating it too! To add hydration to your diet, incorporate foods with high water content - this could include strawberries at breakfast, a cucumber salad at lunch and an apple for an afternoon snack. These water-rich foods not only help quench your thirst but also bring an array of vital nutrients to your plate.

Limit dehydrating drinks: Reduce the intake of drinks that can contribute to dehydration

Dehydrating drinks, like caffeine-rich teas, coffee, and certain fizzy drinks, can counteract your hydration efforts, so be mindful of what you are drinking. When reaching for a drink, opt for water or hydrating alternatives like herbal teas. If you enjoy coffee or tea, try to balance each cup with an additional glass of water. By making these simple switches, you can improve your hydration and control your blood sugars more effectively.

Consistent intake: Instead of drinking large volumes at once, aim for consistent hydration throughout the day

Perhaps set a reminder on your phone or computer to take a few sips every 30 minutes, as this not only helps in keeping dehydration at bay but also avoids the discomfort of consuming large amounts in one go. Over time, this regular intake will become second nature.

Monitor fluid loss: After vigorous exercise or on a particularly hot day, ensure you replace the fluids lost through perspiration
When you have had a workout or it is a hot day, you will naturally sweat more. This means your body is losing precious fluids and therefore staying on top of your hydration becomes even more important. Carrying a reusable water bottle can be handy, helping you gauge how much you are drinking. It is not just about quenching your thirst, but ensuring your body has what it needs to function optimally.

Listen to your body: Thirst is an innate signal. Respond to it promptly
Whenever you feel that gentle nudge of thirst, do not delay; have a sip of water. Keep a water bottle close by, whether at your desk, in your bag, or by your bedside. Over time, tuning into these subtle cues and acting on them promptly can become second nature. It is a simple yet impactful step in ensuring you remain hydrated.

Quality over quantity: While keeping hydrated is important, overhydration can also pose risks
Rather than consuming vast amounts of water quickly, aim to drink little and often and adjust based on your activity level and the climate. Not all fluids are created equal; pure water or natural infusions are ideal choices. Regularly monitoring the colour of your urine can offer a helpful visual guide: a pale straw hue indicates good hydration.

>> ACTION POINTS - PRIORITY 2 <<

Use visual reminders: Keep a bottle of water within reach as a reminder to drink regularly

Make this a seamless part of your daily routine by picking a water bottle you enjoy and keeping it in a visible spot, like your desk or bedside table. Each time you spot the bottle, take a few sips. Over time, this will become a natural habit, ensuring you drink more water throughout the day.

Infusions: If plain water is not appealing, herbal infusions or water flavoured naturally with slices of fruits can be a refreshing alternative

Add slices of your favourite fruits like cucumber, strawberries, or lemon to a jug of water and let it sit for a few hours. Alternatively, herbal teas, such as peppermint or chamomile, can offer a calming, caffeine-free option. These natural additions not only enhance taste but can also make the act of drinking water feel enjoyable.

Alcohol

Alcohol can affect blood sugar levels in unpredictable ways. Some alcoholic drinks contain sugars that can increase glucose, but alcohol itself can lower blood sugar. If consumed on an empty stomach, alcohol heightens the risk of blood sugar levels dropping dangerously low.

As alcohol is technically a toxin, when you consume it, your liver prioritises detoxifying the body of the alcohol over its normal functions. This includes releasing stored glucose in response to low blood sugar, and this can lead to low blood sugars. As well as affecting blood sugar levels and causing more work for the liver, many alcoholic drinks are also very calorie dense, and their regular consumption can cause weight gain.

Alcohol can affect diabetes medication, making them less effective or causing unpredictable changes in their effects. This can be especially dangerous for those on medication that increase insulin levels.

Chronic alcohol consumption can worsen diabetic neuropathy, damaging the nerves in the hands and feet, which can lead on to other serious complications, including infections and foot and lower leg amputation.

Beyond the effects on blood sugar levels, excessive alcohol consumption can have a profound effect on the rest of your body, including:

- liver damage (alcoholic fatty liver disease, hepatitis, and cirrhosis)
- heart problems (irregular heartbeat, a weakening of the heart muscle, increased risk of heart attack, and stroke)
- increased risk of certain types of cancer (mouth, throat, oesophageal, liver, breast, and colorectal)
- causing mental health issues (depression and anxiety)
- brain damage (memory problems and cognitive impairment)
- pancreatitis
- a weakened immune system
- digestive issues (gastritis and ulcers)

The UK guidelines for alcohol consumption are to not drink over 14 units per week, and these 14 units should be spread out over at least 3 days. If you are drinking over this amount and regularly, then perhaps it is a good time to reflect on and work towards moderating your alcohol consumption.

Wine	11% ABV Wine	14% ABV Wine	Beer	3.8% ABV Lager	5.2% ABV Lager
125ml glass	1.4 units	1.8 units	284ml (1/2 pint)	1.1 units	1.5 units
175ml glass	1.9 units	2.4 units	440ml can	1.7 units	2.3 units
250ml glass	2.8 units	3.5 units	568ml pint	2.2 units	3 units
750ml bottle	8.2 units	10.5 units	660ml bottle	2.5 units	3.4 units

>> ACTION POINTS - PRIORITY 1 <<

Reflect on consumption: Before your next drink, take a moment to reflect on its impact on your health

Before raising that glass, take a moment. Think about how alcohol fits into your health journey, especially if you are trying to control your blood sugar levels. Thinking about the impact on things like sugar and insulin can lead to healthier decisions. It is not about denying yourself but making informed choices and when you understand the broader picture; it is easier to opt for moderation or non-alcoholic alternatives.

Educate yourself: Understand how different drinks can affect your blood sugar levels

Learning about the impact of different alcoholic drinks on blood sugar is valuable. If you're aware that combining spirits and sugary soft drinks can cause a spike in blood sugar, you might opt for healthier mixers or alternatives. Knowledge can make all the difference in choosing drinks that align better with your health goals.

>> ACTION POINTS - PRIORITY 2 <<

Embrace alternatives: Experiment with non-alcoholic drinks

On your next shopping trip or evening out, be curious and try non-alcoholic versions of your favourite drink. Delve into the world of mocktails, herbal teas, flavoured sparkling waters, or perhaps some alcohol-free wines, beers, or spirits.

Journal your observations: If you choose to consume alcohol, note its effects on your blood sugar and wellbeing

Every time you have a drink, jot down the type and quantity and then observe how you feel in the hours that follow. Do you notice any changes in your energy, mood, or blood sugar levels? Over time, these notes will paint a clearer picture of how alcohol influences your body.

Artificial Sweeteners

There has been an increase in the popularity and choice of artificial sweeteners in recent years, to combat the growing issue of excessive sugar consumption. On the face of it, there seems to be some logic behind switching from sugar to artificial sweeteners and getting that 'sweetness-hit' without the calories.

Sweetness without sugar - the perfect solution. That must make artificial sweeteners the perfect alternative to sugar? Well, hold that thought for a moment. We will come back to that, as it is an important issue.

Let us first look at some of the more commonly available sweeteners:
- **Sucralose:** A chlorinated derivative of sucrose (white table sugar), sucralose is up to 600 times sweeter than table sugar.
- **Stevia:** A natural sweetener derived from the stevia plant native to Brazil and Paraguay.
- **Aspartame:** A widely used artificial sweetener, aspartame has been linked to a range of health controversies, not the least of which is cancer.
- **Saccharin:** Discovered in the late 19th century, saccharin was the first artificial sweetener.
- **Xylitol:** A sugar alcohol that is found in plants.
- **Erythritol:** A sugar alcohol.

- **Acesulfame Potassium (Ace-K):** Acesulfame potassium is often combined with other sweeteners, including sucralose and aspartame, because of its bitter aftertaste.
- **Agave Nectar:** Although it is promoted as a natural sweetener, agave nectar has a high fructose content and is often very highly processed - bringing it into the realms of 'artificial'.

Beyond adding sweetness to your cup of tea or coffee, artificial sweeteners can negatively affect health in the following ways:

The human body has a reward system that naturally associates sweet taste with calorie content. Consuming something sweet signals the body to expect a caloric intake and when the sweet tastebud receptors are activated, your body triggers the metabolic processes it feels it will need to deal with the expected sugar. Artificial sweeteners, being generally calorie and sugar free, disrupt and upset this process. Over time, this can lead to increased food intake, as the body seeks the calories it has been conditioned to expect from sweet tastes.

Some artificial sweeteners do have a negative effect on insulin, and just because they are calorie-free does not mean that they are healthy. Certain sweeteners (including sucralose and saccharine) can stimulate insulin release and mimic sugar - and continued insulin spikes (triggered by artificial sweeteners) can lead to increased fat storage and insulin resistance.

As noted in the section on fibre, your gut bacteria (your 'microbiome') plays an important role in your health and the function of your immune system. Some artificial sweeteners have been shown to alter the composition of gut bacteria, which has the potential to lead on to a range of health issues, including glucose intolerance and compromised immunity. A disrupted microbiome can also affect nutrient absorption and inflammation levels in the gut, which themselves are linked to obesity and metabolic issues.

Consistent exposure to intensely sweet flavours can heighten your 'sweetness threshold', making naturally sweet foods (like fruit) seem less sweet in comparison. This can lead to an increased dependence on artificially sweetened or sugary foods to satisfy cravings, perpetuating a cycle of sweet addiction (refer back to the section on the 'sugar addiction cycle'). Artificial sweeteners can keep you stuck in that sugar addiction cycle.

When an individual knows they are consuming low-calorie, artificially sweetened foods or drinks, they might feel it is okay to eat more later. This is known as "dietary compensation" and can inadvertently lead to increased caloric intake throughout the day.

An issue to not be overlooked is that certain artificial sweeteners can break down into metabolites (substances produced during metabolism) in the body. Aspartame, for example, can degrade into methanol, which can then convert into formaldehyde (a chemical often used in the process of embalming) - which is toxic.

Excessive consumption of artificial sweeteners has been linked to other health concerns, including migraines, cardiovascular diseases and certain types of cancers.

>> ACTION POINTS - PRIORITY 1 <<

Read labels carefully: Ensure you are not only looking at the sugar content but also checking for artificial sweeteners
When shopping, take a moment to study the ingredients list on the back of the packaging. While the 'sugar-free' label might catch your eye, dig deeper to spot names like aspartame, saccharin, or sucralose. These are common artificial sweeteners.

Rethink your drink: Evaluate your drink choices and reduce your intake of drinks containing artificial sweeteners
Next time you are thirsty, take a moment to consider your drink. Are you reaching for a drink laden with artificial sweeteners? Perhaps it is a diet cola or flavoured water? Swap these out for more natural options like plain water, herbal teas, or drinks with no added sweeteners. Over time, your taste buds will adjust.

Limit Processed Foods: The fewer processed items in your diet, the less likely you will inadvertently consume artificial sweeteners
Next time you shop, gravitate towards fresh fruits, veggies, grains, and lean proteins. These foods, in their natural state, are free from added sweeteners. Opting for homemade snacks and meals avoids hidden

artificial additives and lets you enjoy natural flavours.

>> ACTION POINT - PRIORITY 2 <<

Embrace natural: Try natural alternatives for sweetness and always in moderation

If you want a sweet taste without artificial ingredients, try using honey in small amounts as a natural alternative. Gradually, adopting natural sweeteners means opting for a healthier alternative and experiencing the real flavours of food.

Sodium

When we look at the nutritional information found on the back of food packaging, we frequently overlook sodium. Found naturally, this mineral is commonly connected to salt and has a big impact on blood sugar control and overall health.

Sodium is one of the primary electrolytes in the body and is often mistaken for salt. Salt (sodium chloride) comprises about 40% sodium and 60% chloride. Sodium helps maintain fluid balance, influences muscle function, and is vital for nerve transmission.

Though essential, like everything, it is about maintaining balance. Whilst the body is efficient at maintaining a state called homeostasis (the process by which the body maintains a stable internal environment to ensure optimal functioning of its systems), through your diet you can negatively influence those systems and create problems. Too much sodium can be an issue, as elevated sodium intake has been linked to high blood pressure, which then increases the risk of cardiovascular disease. Type 2 diabetes already increases the risk of heart problems and there is emerging research that suggests that excessive sodium might impair the body's insulin sensitivity.

>> ACTION POINTS - PRIORITY 1 <<

Review your hydration routine: Establish a daily water-drinking routine to ensure you are flushing out excess sodium

Staying well-hydrated is a straightforward way to help manage sodium levels. To cultivate this healthy habit, start every day with a glass of water. Find a reusable bottle you like, fill it up and keep it with you during the day. Set reminders on your phone or stick post-it notes in visible places as gentle nudges. If plain water does not appeal, infuse it with slices of fresh fruit or cucumber for a refreshing twist.

Choose fresh over processed: Fresh foods contain less sodium than their processed counterparts

Begin by buying fresh vegetables, fruits and unprocessed cuts of meat - and gradually phase out pre-packaged, canned or frozen items (especially those with a lengthy ingredient list). Embracing fresh foods not only helps limit sodium but also enriches your meals with natural flavours.

>> ACTION POINTS - PRIORITY 2 <<

Look in your food cupboard: Check sodium content on packaged foods and consider healthier alternatives

Start with a scan of your food cupboard and look at the nutrition labels on your packaged foods - paying attention to the sodium content. If it seems high, make a list and next time you shop, explore alternatives with lower sodium. Fresh herbs, spices, or a squeeze of lemon can offer flavourful substitutes to sodium-heavy products.

Cook at home: Preparing meals at home gives you control over the sodium and seasoning, allowing for better sodium management
Start by setting aside specific days or evenings for cooking. Equip your kitchen with a range of herbs and spices, allowing you to experiment with flavours without relying on sodium. Refer to cookbooks or online platforms for inspiration.

Mind your condiments: Sauces and condiments can be significant sodium contributors
When choosing condiments, make it a habit to glance at the label, particularly the sodium content. Whether it is ketchup, soy sauce, or salad dressing, these can sometimes be saltier than you might expect. Perhaps find lower-sodium alternatives or even try making your own versions at home with reduced salt. Remember, it is not about sacrificing taste; it is about embracing a healthier balance.

Taste before you season: Before automatically adding salt, taste your food
The next time you are about to sprinkle salt on your dish, pause and take a bite first. Savour the flavours. You may discover that your meal already tastes fine, or perhaps only a tiny pinch of salt is needed. By making this simple change, you are not only reducing your sodium intake, but also becoming more attuned to the tastes of your food.

Portion Sizes

The shift towards ever-increasing portion sizes presents an enormous problem in our modern-day society. The growing number of non-communicable diseases is likely attributed to aggressive marketing campaigns and changing societal norms that promote overconsumption and weight gain.

When you are trying to prevent or reverse type 2 diabetes, monitoring portion sizes is an important consideration - remember... is it not just about what you eat, but also how much of it you eat too.

Blood sugar levels increase directly in response to not just what is eaten, but also to the amount of food eaten too (refer back to the section on glycaemic index and glycaemic load). When you eat larger portions, your bloodstream receives a larger influx of glucose. The pancreas then produces insulin to help cells absorb this glucose, but over time these consistently large portion sizes can lead to excessive demands on the pancreas, making it work it harder, reducing its efficacy and contributing to insulin resistance.

Overeating, even with healthy foods, can lead to weight gain, high blood sugar, and digestive problems.

Understanding standard serving sizes (like recognising that a serving of cooked vegetables typically mirrors the size of a fist) can be helpful. Simple changes, such as using smaller plates or adhering to the 'Half Plate Rule' (half vegetables, a quarter protein, and a quarter complex carbohydrates) can also encourage better portion control.

Being in tune with your body's signals of fullness, avoiding distractions during meals (mindful eating, which we will cover later), and keeping a food diary can offer useful insights. It is also good to recognise the emotional aspects tied to your eating habits, whether they be stress or joy, as they can all prompt overeating.

>> ACTION POINTS - PRIORITY 1 <<

Educate yourself: Familiarise yourself with standard serving sizes to ensure you are consuming appropriate amounts
Start by looking at the back of your food packages and look for the information on the recommended serving size. Alternatively, invest in a handy portion control guide or look online for visuals that compare food portions to everyday objects (for instance, a serving of meat is often likened to the size of a deck of cards). As you become more familiar with these guidelines, it will better equip you to serve up just the right amount.

Plate strategy: Use the half plate rule as a guide for balanced meals

Embrace the half plate rule for well-balanced meals - when serving up, visualise your plate divided into thirds and fill one half with vegetables or salad with the remaining half, split equally (one quarter for proteins like lean meat, fish or beans and the last quarter for complex carbohydrates like whole grains or starchy vegetables). This simple visual guide ensures you are getting a nourishing mix of foods, promoting better blood sugar control and health.

Stay hydrated: Drink water before meals to assist with satiety

To help manage your appetite, make a gentle habit of sipping a glass of water about 10-15 minutes before eating. This simple step can make you feel fuller, potentially reducing the amount you eat. Not only does it aid in hydration, but it is a natural and easy way to cue your body, preparing it for the meal ahead.

>> ACTION POINTS - PRIORITY 2 <<

Mindful eating: Practice being present during meals

To practice mindful eating, begin by eliminating distractions - put away your phone, turn off the TV and sit down at a table. As you eat, focus on the flavours, textures and aromas of your food. Chew slowly, allowing yourself to truly taste every bite. By giving your meal your full attention, you will naturally tune into your body's signals, helping you recognise when you are comfortably full.

Emotional check: Recognise and address any emotional triggers that might lead to overeating

Addressing emotional triggers is key to understanding overeating patterns, so begin by pausing for a moment before eating (especially if you are not truly hungry). Ask yourself, "what am I feeling right now?" It might be stress, loneliness, or even joy. Once identified, consider healthier coping strategies (like a short walk, deep breathing exercises, or chatting with a friend). By building this self-awareness, you are equipping yourself to make better choices, not just in food, but in how you respond to your emotions.

Food diary: Consider maintaining a food diary to monitor your eating patterns

Starting a food diary is a useful way to become more aware of your eating habits. Grab a small notebook or use a digital app and jot down everything you eat and drink throughout the day. It does not need to be overly detailed (a brief note on what and roughly how much you had will do). Over time, this record can offer surprising insights into your portion sizes and eating patterns, allowing you to recognise areas to adjust.

Calories and Weight Management

Calories are simply units of energy. Think of them as the fuel your body needs to function – from performing daily tasks to ensuring that your heart beats and you continue to breathe. Food and drink provide you with this energy, and you get calories from three macronutrients: carbohydrates, proteins and fats.

Each of these has a specific caloric value:

Carbohydrates: 4 calories per gram
Proteins: 4 calories per gram
Fats: 9 calories per gram

When we consider the fluctuations in our own weight, it is important to understand that it is a balance between biochemistry and physics. When you consume more calories than you expend, your body stores the surplus in your fat cells. Over time, consistent caloric surplus can result in weight gain. Conversely, where you burn more than you consume, your body is forced to utilise your fat reserves, which then leads to weight loss.

The law of conservation of energy states that energy can neither be created nor destroyed - only converted from one form of energy to another.

It is important to understand that the source of calories play an important role too, as whole foods not only provide nutrients and sustained energy, but they also help to keep blood sugar levels stable. Consuming ultra-processed foods might not fill you up (calorie-dense and nutrient deficient), which can lead to overeating - even if you have already met your caloric needs.

Excess weight, particularly visceral fat around the abdomen, is associated with insulin resistance, and increases the risk of developing type 2 diabetes. Foods most associated with weight gain, notably ultra-processed ones high in sugars and unhealthy fats, can also disrupt blood sugar management. Therefore, effective weight management in the prevention or reversal of type 2 diabetes must be an important consideration.

>> ACTION POINTS - PRIORITY 1 <<

Work out your Basal Metabolic Rate (BMR) to establish your daily calorie needs and then keep a food diary to help you either stay within that amount to maintain your weight, or create an intentional calorie deficit to help you lose weight

Understanding your daily calorie needs is key to managing your weight. Your BMR is the number of calories your body needs at rest. To calculate it, use an online BMR calculator where you can enter age, gender, height, weight and average activity levels. Once you have your BMR, track what you eat with a food diary. To maintain weight, eat around your BMR in calories; to lose weight, aim for less (a 300-500kcals per day deficit might be good to aim for). Remember, the quality of the calories you consume matters just as much as the quantity, so focus on nutritious choices for better health.

Try to balance the calories on your plate
I am all for balance with the three macronutrients, not favouring one over the others. Using an online food diary app, start by recording everything in your evening meal.

From the diary data, look at the amount (in grams) of the carbohydrate, protein and fats in your meal, and then work these out as a percentage (for example, a 625kcal meal might be made up of 45g of complex carbohydrates (180kcals (45g x 4kcal per gram)), 55g of protein (220kcals (55g x 4kcal per gram)) and 25g of healthy fats (225kcals (25g x 9kcals per gram)).

This would represent a well-balanced meal, with 29% being carbohydrates, 35% being protein, and 36% being fat.

Meal balancing can take a little bit of practice, but becomes easier with time.

Reflect on your typical daily meals. Are they nutrient-dense or empty calories?
Record all your food and drink intake for a week. Analyse each item: does it contain vitamins, minerals, and other beneficial nutrients, or is

it mainly providing calories with little nutritional value? Prioritise foods that nourish your body, such as colourful vegetables, lean proteins and whole grains.

Aim to incorporate at least 30 minutes of movement into your day
Start by setting aside specific times in your day, perhaps a 30-minute walk after meals or taking the stairs instead of the lift. Dancing to your favourite songs, gardening, or even stretching during TV ad breaks counts too. Consistency is vital. As these activities become part of your routine, you will naturally discover more ways to stay active and enhance weight management and blood sugar control.

Stay hydrated: Drinking water can not only help with metabolism but also ensures you do not mistake thirst for hunger
Keep a refillable water bottle by your side throughout the day to remind you to drink regularly. Before reaching for a snack, have a glass of water and wait a few minutes. Sometimes, hunger can be confused with thirst and so by ensuring you are well-hydrated, you will better discern true hunger cues - helping in making mindful eating decisions and keeping the calories in check.

Practice reading food labels the next time you shop
Next time you are shopping, take a moment to inspect the food labels of your favourite foods. Look for the calorie count per serving and note down the portion size. Glance at the list of ingredients; shorter lists often signify less processing. Getting to know these labels will help you understand what you are consuming and make better choices.

Experiment with portion sizes during meals, listening to your body's cues

When serving your meals, begin with slightly smaller portions than usual and as you eat, pay close attention to your body's signals. Are you still hungry or just eating out of habit? If you are still hungry after finishing, it might be okay to have a little more. Over time, you will become more attuned to your body's genuine hunger and fullness cues. By adjusting portions and listening to your body, you will naturally find the right balance that supports both satisfaction and weight management.

Examine your diet: How balanced is your plate during meals?

Take a moment at your next mealtime to assess your plate visually. Ideally, half should be filled with colourful vegetables (think broccoli, carrots, or spinach), a quarter with lean protein (fish, chicken, tofu, or beans) and the remaining quarter with whole grains (quinoa, brown rice, or perhaps red lentil pasta). This ensures a mix of essential nutrients. If your plate does not quite match up, consider adding some veggies or swapping out white rice for quinoa. By paying attention to this balance, you are not just counting calories, but making every calorie count towards nourishing your body.

Limit empty calories: Foods and drinks that provide calories with little nutritional value can quickly lead to weight gain

Reducing empty calories is a game-changer for weight and health. Start by being more conscious when you are thirsty; choose water, herbal tea, or unsweetened beverages over sugary drinks. When hungry, choose homemade meals and snacks where you can. Swapping out that packet of crisps for a handful of nuts or choosing a piece of fruit over a chocolate bar, can make a world of difference.

>> ACTION POINTS - PRIORITY 2 <<

Emotional check: Recognise and address any emotional triggers that might lead to overeating
Addressing emotional triggers is key to understanding overeating patterns, so begin by pausing for a moment before eating (especially if you are not truly hungry). Ask yourself, "what am I feeling right now?" It might be stress, loneliness, or even joy. Once identified, consider healthier coping strategies (like a short walk, deep breathing exercises, or chatting with a friend). By building this self-awareness, you are equipping yourself to make better choices, not just in food, but in how you respond to your emotions.

Embrace home cooking where possible, giving you control over ingredients and portion sizes and diabetes prevention
Start with one home-cooked meal a week, using fresh ingredients. Choose simple recipes initially and gradually expand your repertoire. As you cook, you decide what goes in, allowing you to favour natural, whole foods and manage portion sizes.

Intermittent Fasting

I am a fan of intermittent fasting, as it was (and still is) one of my go-to tools for controlling my weight and my blood sugars.

In recent times, intermittent fasting has grown in popularity and, when used correctly and under guidance (at least to begin with), intermittent fasting could also be a beneficial tool for you, too.

It is important to understand that intermittent fasting is NOT 'dieting', nor is it 'starvation' (as some people may think), but it is simply a pattern of eating. It divides your day into periods of eating and not eating - giving your digestive system a well-deserved break, and your body the chance to use its stored glucose (glycogen) and fats. Extended periods without food can also help your body be more responsive to insulin, which can help to control your blood sugar levels. Intermittent fasting also encourages a process called autophagy (where your body breaks old cells down, recycling damaged components and removing debris - to help maintain their proper function).

While several variations of intermittent fasting exist, these are the two most common methods that I see being used today:

The 24-hour fast

As the name suggests, this method involves abstaining from food and caloric drinks for 24 consecutive hours. As an example: if you have your last meal at 7pm on Monday, you will resume eating at 7 pm on Tuesday. During the fasting period, you consume adequate amounts of water, herbal teas, or black coffee (without sugar or sweeteners). It is not recommended to do 24-hour fasts consecutively or more than once per week.

The 18:6 Fast

This method involves fasting for 18 hours and eating (healthily and not to excess) during a 6-hour window. As an example: your eating window could be from 12pm to 8pm. This might mean skipping breakfast and eating your meals between 1pm and 7pm. Again, water intake must be maintained, and you can also drink other mostly non-caloric drinks like herbal teas or black coffee. If you find the 18:6 method preferable, it can be done more frequently than once a week, if that works for you.

Whichever method you choose, please find enjoyment in the process and do not make it feel tedious or a chore. If you learn to enjoy intermittent fasting, the way it makes you feel and the benefits it brings, you are more likely to incorporate it into your routine - not just in the short term, but for many years to come.

As with any significant change in routine, it would be remiss of me not to offer you some precautions and considerations when it comes to intermittent fasting:

- If you have type 2 diabetes and are considering intermittent fasting (especially if you are on medication) it is important to consult with your doctor or nutritionist first.
- During intermittent fasting periods, it is crucial that you remain hydrated. Water, herbal teas and unsweetened black coffee/tea are good.
- When you eat after your fast, focus on nutrient-dense whole foods that support your energy and nutritional needs. This is not a time for calorie-dense, nutrient-poor processed foods. Also, do not over-eat to compensate for the missed meal(s).
- Blood sugar monitoring during fasting periods can provide you with useful information about how the fast affects your blood glucose levels.
- If you have never tried intermittent fasting before, you might want to begin with shorter periods and gradually extend, as you monitor your body's response to it.

While there are many benefits to intermittent fasting, it is not for everyone. Some may experience adverse effects or find it challenging to adhere to, and it is important to seek guidance before starting.

>> ACTION POINTS - PRIORITY 1 <<

Educate yourself: Before embarking on intermittent fasting, familiarise yourself with its principles and potential impact

Understand its benefits and potential challenges (this will allow you to make informed decisions tailored to your health and whether intermittent fasting is right for you). Consider consulting with a nutritionist to ensure this approach aligns with your health goals.

Start slowly: If new to fasting, begin with shorter periods and see how your body responds before attempting longer fasts

Take it gently to start with. Begin by introducing shorter fasts, perhaps skipping just one meal, or extending the time between dinner and breakfast. Then maybe progress on to an 18:6 fast and then once you are accustomed to that, then on to a full 24-hour fast. Tune into your body's signals and notice how you feel, your energy levels and any changes in your blood sugars. By easing into it with an 18:6 fast, you will give your body the chance to adapt, and you can then decide if longer fasting periods feel right for you.

Stay hydrated: Throughout fasting periods, keep up with water or non-caloric drink intake

During intermittent fasting, it is essential to keep your body hydrated - even if you are skipping meals, do not skip on fluids. Regularly sip on water throughout the day. If plain water feels bland, you can also opt for herbal teas or infusions, which add a hint of flavour with no calories. Black tea or black coffee (without sugar!) is also okay. Regular fluid intake not only keeps you hydrated but can also aid in curbing hunger pangs.

Monitor responses: Monitor blood sugar levels, energy levels and overall wellbeing

Regularly check your blood sugar levels using a reliable glucose monitor, especially if you have type 2 diabetes. Also, note how you feel energy-wise and mentally throughout the day. Any drastic changes or prolonged discomfort may be a signal to reassess or tweak your fasting approach. If you struggle during a fasting period, bring it to a close at that point and revisit it again the following week.

Nutrient density: Include nutrient-dense foods in your eating windows for optimal nutrition.

During your eating windows with intermittent fasting, it is essential to maximise the nutrients you consume. Choose whole foods rich in vitamins, minerals, and fibre, such as leafy greens, colourful vegetables, lean proteins, and whole grains. Make sure not to compensate for the calories omitted during the day by consuming a larger evening meal. Keep your evening meal the same size and calorie value as a normal day.

Reassess and adjust: If you find a particular method challenging, consider trying another or adjusting your eating and fasting windows

Intermittent fasting is not a one-size-fits-all approach. If you are finding your current method tough, it is okay to re-evaluate. Maybe an 18-hour fasting window feels too long; try reducing it to 14 hours. If evening fasting is not for you, consider fasting in the morning. The key is to find a balance that suits your body and lifestyle, ensuring you manage your blood sugars effectively.

The Dawn Phenomenon

If you are pre-diabetic or type 2 diabetic, you may have noticed that your morning blood sugar readings are higher than they were before you went to sleep. Without knowing why, this can be worrying, a little confusing and even disheartening. Worry not - as a normal process, called the 'Dawn Phenomenon', causes this early morning rise.

Everyone, not just those with type 2 diabetes, experiences the Dawn Phenomenon. Between 2am and 8am, your body releases several hormones - including cortisol, glucagon, growth hormone and epinephrine. These hormones form part of the body's natural waking-up process, helping to provide you with the energy needed to start the day when you awaken.

The problem is that these hormones can also reduce your cell's sensitivity to insulin, which then results in a rise in blood sugar levels. While this hormone cocktail is surging through your bloodstream, your liver can add to the rise by producing a surge of additional glucose (called gluconeogenesis).

The pancreas then responds to this rise in glucose levels by producing extra insulin and, for someone without type 2 diabetes, this brings the blood glucose levels back down and keeps them stable. For pre-diabetics and type 2 diabetics, however, this additional insulin either is not produced in sufficient quantities or the body does not respond to it as efficiently, resulting in the elevated blood glucose levels - causing the Dawn Phenomenon.

Understanding and addressing the Dawn Phenomenon is important, as morning hyperglycaemia (raised blood sugars) can set the pattern for the rest of your day - which can make blood glucose control more challenging.

>> ACTION POINTS - PRIORITY 1 <<

Monitor and document: Regularly checking blood glucose levels at bedtime, during the night (around 3am) and at waking can help determine if you are experiencing the Dawn Phenomenon
To monitor and understand the Dawn Phenomenon:

- **Bedtime:** *Before you go to sleep, use a blood glucose monitor to check your blood sugar levels. Record the reading in a journal or a diabetes app.*
- **Around 3am:** *Set an alarm to wake up around 3am and check your blood glucose levels again. Record this reading as well.*
- **Morning:** *As soon as you wake up, before eating or drinking anything, check your blood sugar once more and note it down.*

By consistently tracking your blood sugars at these times, you will identify any patterns of rising blood sugar levels in the morning - which can then be shared with your doctor.

Adjust meal timing: Some find that a small, healthy snack before bed can stabilise blood sugar levels

To address the Dawn Phenomenon with adjusted meal timing:

- ***Snack selection:*** *Choose a small, balanced snack before bedtime. Opt for options rich in protein or healthy fats, like a handful of almonds, Greek yogurt, or a slice of whole grain toast with peanut butter.*
- ***Moderation:*** *Keep the portion size small to avoid overeating. This will help stabilise blood glucose levels through the night.*
- ***Consistency:*** *Make this a nightly routine to establish consistency, as over time, it can contribute to more stable morning blood sugar levels.*

Review medications: If you are on diabetes medication, consult your doctor about when you take them

To optimise your medication for the Dawn Phenomenon:

- ***Speak with your doctor to discuss your medication timing:*** *Share your concerns about morning blood sugar spikes.*
- ***Follow professional guidance:*** *Your doctor will provide recommendations for changing the timing of your diabetes medication to suit your specific needs.*
- ***Regular Monitoring:*** *After implementing any changes, continue to monitor your blood sugar levels at various times, including in the morning, to ensure the adjustments are effective.*

>> ACTION POINTS - PRIORITY 2 <<

Avoid Alcohol: Alcohol can interfere with the liver's glucose production

To reduce the impact of alcohol on the Dawn Phenomenon:

- *__Evening abstinence:__ Choose not to consume alcohol in the evening, especially close to your bedtime.*
- *__Moderation:__ If you consume alcohol, do so in moderation and avoid excessive amounts or heavy drinking.*
- *__Hydration:__ Ensure you are well-hydrated, drinking water alongside alcohol, to minimise its effects on blood sugar levels.*

Stay active: Incorporate evening physical activities

After your evening meal, instead of being sitting down in front of the tv, go out for a leisurely 20-minute walk. It is a simple way to stay active with no strenuous exercise. This post-dinner activity can help regulate blood sugar levels, potentially reducing the impact of the Dawn Phenomenon.

Relax and unwind: Dedicate at least 15 minutes before bed to stress-reducing activities

Try to create a relaxing pre-bedtime routine. Dedicate 15 minutes to unwind before you go to sleep. Choose activities that calm your mind and reduce stress (such as reading, meditation, or deep breathing exercises). Regularly practicing this technique can reduce the impact of the Dawn Phenomenon by regulating your body's stress response.

The Somogyi Effect

The Somogyi Effect, discovered by Dr. Michael Somogyi, is a condition where blood sugars drop at night and are elevated in the morning.

Interestingly, this surge is not a straightforward response to what was eaten the day before or perhaps to missed medication - it is the body's defence mechanism against dangerously low blood sugar levels.

The Somogyi Effect begins with a period of low blood sugar during the night, and this can be caused by one of many reasons - such as taking too much medication in the evening, perhaps not having a substantial enough evening snack, or increased physical activity the previous day.

When blood sugar drops to low levels, the body acts and it releases stress hormones, which include cortisol and glucagon. These hormones encourage the liver to release stored glucose - this is a completely natural defence mechanism, ensuring the body has enough glucose to function properly. The potential problem arises in those with type 2 diabetes, as the body might overcompensate, leading to an excessive release of glucose. By morning, this results in high blood sugar levels, a rebound response to the night-time low.

The most common cause of the Somogyi Effect is related to insulin (if long-acting insulin is taken in the evening, it might cause a drop in blood sugar levels during sleep) or other diabetes medication. Missing or having a light evening meal, especially after taking medication, can also trigger the Somogyi Effect too - when the body does not have enough glucose from food, causing an eventual dip in levels. Engaging in strenuous physical activity, especially later in the day, can increase insulin sensitivity ("not a bad thing", you might reasonably think). This does, however, mean that the same dose of diabetes medication might have a stronger effect, dropping blood glucose levels more than expected.

Alcohol can also be a factor (as it inhibits gluconeogenesis), and therefore, if alcohol is consumed in the evening without adequate food, it can lead to night-time hypoglycaemia.

Some symptoms of night-time lows blood sugar levels include:
- Night sweats or waking up with damp sheets.
- Morning headaches.
- Disturbed sleep or nightmares.
- Feeling unusually tired upon waking, despite seemingly adequate sleep.
- Unexplained elevated blood sugar levels in the morning.

While the most obvious sign of the Somogyi Effect is a high morning blood sugar reading, without the corresponding evidence of night-time hypoglycaemia, it can be challenging to diagnose and can be mistaken for the Dawn Phenomenon. Continuous Glucose Monitoring units (CGM's) or a timed blood sugar check during the night can offer better insight as to what is happening while you are asleep.

>> ACTION POINTS - PRIORITY 1 <<

Consistent monitoring: Recognising the pattern is the first step
Consistent monitoring is the key to addressing the Somogyi Effect - so invest in a Continuous Glucose Monitoring (CGM) machine or set alarms to wake up and check your blood sugar levels during the night. This will help you understand your specific blood sugar patterns that are occurring while you sleep - allowing you (and your doctor) to make informed adjustments to your diabetes medication plan. By pinpointing the cause of morning highs, you can take steps to achieve better blood sugar control.

Dietary re-evaluation: An evening snack, rich in protein and healthy fats, can provide sustained glucose release during the night
Dietary adjustments can help combat the Somogyi Effect, so consider having a nighttime snack consisting of protein and healthy fats (e.g. a handful of nuts or Greek yogurt with berries). These choices promote a sustained release of glucose during the night, helping to stabilise your blood sugar levels.

Physical activity: While staying active is essential, it might be beneficial to move intense workouts to earlier in the day, or perhaps reduce evening medication doses on days when you are very active

Incorporating physical activity into your routine to manage the Somogyi Effect is crucial. Choose moderate activities like an evening walk or gentle stretching. If you engage in intense workouts, consider scheduling them earlier in the day to reduce the risk of nighttime lows. On days when you are very active, discuss potential medication adjustments with your doctor, as reducing evening doses may be necessary.

Limit evening alcohol: If consuming alcohol, pair it with a meal or a substantial snack to prevent sudden drops in blood sugar levels

To limit the impact of evening alcohol on your blood sugar levels and address the Somogyi Effect, consider these steps:

- **Plan your alcohol consumption**: If you choose to have alcohol in the evening, do so in moderation and always pair it with a healthy meal or substantial snack.
- **Choose wisely:** Opt for drinks with lower sugar content (such as dry wines or spirits and avoid sugary mixers or cocktails).
- **Snack smart:** Before bedtime, have a protein and healthy fat-rich snack (like a handful of nuts, Greek yogurt, or a slice of cheese).
- **Monitor effectively:** Keep a record of your blood sugar levels before and after alcohol consumption to identify patterns or issues.

Medication adjustments: It might be beneficial to review your medication with your doctor

To address the Somogyi Effect, take these steps to review your medication effectively:

- ***Schedule an appointment with your doctor:*** *Contact your doctor and request an appointment specifically to discuss your medication in relation to nighttime blood sugar levels.*
- ***Prepare Information:*** *Before your appointment, keep a record of your blood sugar readings, especially those during the night (noting any symptoms or patterns you have observed).*
- ***Open dialogue:*** *During the appointment, express your concerns about nighttime lows and provide the information you have gathered (ask if adjusting your medication, its timing, or dosage could help manage the issue).*
- ***Follow medical guidance:*** *Based on your doctor's recommendations, make any necessary adjustments to your medication routine, and monitor your blood sugar as advised.*

Understanding Food Labels

In supermarkets, you will notice shelf after shelf of colourful packaging, enticing imagery and catchy slogans. Put bluntly, it is little more than a deception, and I encourage you to see beyond the marketing hype and look at the most important part of the packaging - the food label. At first glance, food labels can seem a little daunting but with a little direction, they can become your friend and can certainly help you make healthier food choices.

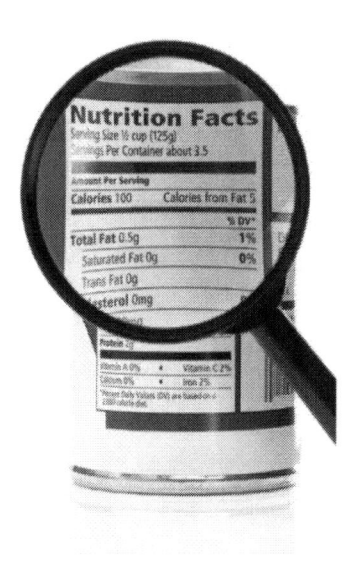

Every packaged product has a label, often on the back or side, and that advises you of what is inside the product, including the ingredients and the nutritional information.

Let us take a quick look at what you can expect to see on a food label:

Ingredients list: Ingredients are listed by quantity, from highest to lowest. If sugars or unhealthy fats appear at the beginning, that is a red flag - avoid.

Serving size and servings per container: All nutritional information on the label pertains to the serving size. Check how many servings are in the entire package, as it is easy to consume multiple servings in one sitting.

Total calories: This gives you an idea of the energy you get from a serving of the food. This is important if you are watching your weight.

Fat: Look for the breakdown of saturated, unsaturated, and trans fats. Prioritise foods with unsaturated fats, limit those with saturated fats and avoid those with trans fats.

Carbohydrates: This is perhaps the most scrutinised area for those with type 2 diabetes. Remember, it is not just about sugars, but the total carbohydrate count that matters.

Sugars: Added sugars can rapidly spike blood sugar levels.

Sodium: Excessive sodium can contribute to high blood pressure.

Fibre: Dietary fibre can help with blood sugar regulation by slowing down the digestion of carbohydrates.

Protein: Proteins are vital for repairing and building tissue.

Vitamins and minerals: Some labels list certain vitamins and minerals. Some of these can be helpful in blood sugar control.

So, we are agreed - food labels offer important and useful information to help you make educated food choices. They are indeed worthy of a deeper dive, so let us inspect these in more detail.

Food Labels - The Ingredients List

The ingredients list shows exactly what is in the food, and understanding the basics can guide you towards making healthier choices.

On any packaged food item (certainly in the UK and many other countries too), the ingredients must be listed in descending order of weight at the time they were used to make the product. This means the first ingredient listed contributes the most by weight to the final product, and the last ingredient the least.

There are certain ingredients that it is wise to be cautious of, and these include:

- **Sugars and sweeteners:** Look out for terms like glucose, fructose, honey, syrup, maltose and other '-ose' endings, as these are often types of sugars. Many processed foods contain significant amounts of hidden sugars, which can negatively impact blood sugar levels (don't forget to download my pocket guide to help you!).
- **Unhealthy fats:** Trans fats and certain saturated fats can elevate cholesterol levels and impact heart health. Ingredients like hydrogenated oils and fats are red flags.

- **Salt:** Listed as sodium chloride, high salt content can contribute to high blood pressure.
- **Additives and preservatives:** You may choose to limit your intake of certain additives, colourings, or preservatives.
- **'E' numbers:** Many food additives are listed with an 'E' followed by a number. This system classifies these ingredients based on their safety assessments. However, not all 'E' numbers are bad, as some are naturally occurring compounds like vitamin C (E300) or beetroot red (E162).

Spotting ingredients you recognise and can pronounce is a good sign. They often show the product is closer to its natural state or certainly closer to resembling 'real' food. Whole foods, or foods that are closer to their natural form, typically contain more beneficial nutrients and fewer additives or preservatives - and often fewer ingredients.

>> ACTION POINTS - PRIORITY 1 <<

Allocate a few minutes during your next shopping trip to carefully read the ingredients lists of the products you frequently consume.
Pause for a moment with each product you are about to place in your basket. Flip it over and scan the ingredients - especially for those items you eat regularly. By familiarising yourself with what is truly inside, you will become more conscious of your choices and better equipped to nourish your body.

Create a cheat sheet of common ingredient names, especially sugars and unhealthy fats, to carry with you or have on your phone

Start by jotting down common aliases for sugars and unhealthy fats, such as 'fructose' or 'hydrogenated oils' (alternatively, please download my 'sugars' guide and save this list on your phone or print it off and pop it in your wallet/purse. When you are shopping, give it a quick glance before you check product labels. This little cheat sheet will help ensure those hidden villains do not slip into your basket.

www.diabetessolutions.co.uk/tkp-bonuspack

Aim to fill most of your basket with foods that have minimal or no ingredient lists, like fresh fruits, vegetables, lean meats and whole grains.

Reach for vibrant fruits, crunchy vegetables, lean meats and whole grains. These wholesome choices rarely come with long ingredient lists or hidden surprises. By focusing on foods in their natural state, you are not only simplifying your shopping, but also enriching your diet with genuine nourishment.

Food Labels - Serving Sizes

The next time you look at a food label, you will probably see the 'servings per container' or sometimes 'servings per pack'. It is important to understand what this means, as what you might consider being a portion or serving might not always align with the thoughts of the manufacturer (and as we will find out in the section on the 'traffic light system', some food companies reduce their so-called 'portion sizes' down to ridiculously small amounts so that they make their food look healthier than it really is).

Let us look at an example - you open a box of breakfast cereal. The label proudly claims it has only 150 calories per serving, which sounds great. You fill your bowl, add the milk and munch away.

However, on closer inspection, those 150 calories are for a serving size of 30g (which is a tiny portion size for an adult) and you have just poured out a heaped bowl without measuring. That means that you could easily consume 3 or 4 times a 'typical' serving size as stated by the manufacturer - 450 to 600 calories - just for breakfast, and that is before you factor in the milk!

Near to the serving size information, you will often find the servings per container or servings per pack information. This denotes the number of servings you can expect within that entire container or pack. To illustrate, on the way to the cinema, you drop into a supermarket and see a 120g bag of popcorn. You take a quick glance at the nutritional information on the back before and you notice it has 150kcals, 20g of carbohydrate and 10g of sugar in it. You buy it and then consume the entire bag whilst watching the film, safe knowing that with just 150kcals in the pack, it is a relatively low-calorie snack.

What you failed to notice was that the figures above were 'per serving' and not for the entire bag. According to the popcorn manufacturer, there are 6 servings in that single bag. That means you have just inadvertently eaten 750kcals, 120g of carbohydrate and - more worryingly - 60g of sugar.

You can see how 'servings per pack' can easily catch you out, especially when a packet might shout about being 'low in sugar' or 'low in fat'. But a closer look at the label might show that to make that claim, the manufacturer had to make the advertised serving size unrealistically small. It is a tactic that they use a lot… don't fall for it!

>> ACTION POINT - PRIORITY 1 <<

Begin at home: For the next week, make it a point to measure out serving sizes for all your meals

For the next week, at every meal, simply take out a measuring cup or kitchen scale and portion out your foods based on the suggested serving sizes. This is not a forever task, but rather a learning exercise. You will be surprised at how different the manufacturer's idea of a serving is from yours. Over time, you will get a better eye for what, say, 30g of steel-cut oats or 100g of red lentil pasta looks like, helping you make more informed choices even when you are not measuring.

>> ACTION POINT - PRIORITY 2 <<

Log and reflect: Write down any surprises or revelations you find about your regular food items

Keeping a small notebook in your kitchen or using a notes app on your phone, jot down any products that surprise you with their serving sizes. For example, if you have always thought half a chocolate bar was one serving, but the label says otherwise, write it down. Over the week, you will gather a list of foods that might have been tricking you into consuming more than you realised.

Food Labels - Total Calories

The 'total calories' section on a food label provides information about the amount of energy 'one serving' of that food provides. However, as we have just seen, it is easy to get misled by 'serving sizes' on food labels as these are determined by the manufacturer, and they might not be a realistic representation of what you might consider being a 'serving'.

Some foods may be calorie-rich but nutrient-poor (as we covered in the section on processed and ultra-processed foods). These are known as 'empty calories'. Foods that are high in sugars, unhealthy fats, and alcohol often fall into this category. Consuming too many empty calories can lead to weight gain and blood sugar spikes, both of which are undesirable.

Armed with an understanding of total calories, you are better positioned to make healthier food choices by matching your caloric intake with your daily energy expenditure (use an online calculator to work this figure out). If you are trying to lose weight, aim for a caloric deficit; consume fewer calories than you burn. Choose foods that offer more nutrients per calorie. Foods rich in vitamins, minerals, and fibre, such as fruits, vegetables, whole grains, and lean proteins are all excellent choices.

Drinks, especially sugary ones and many hot drinks from coffee shops, can be a problem, as they are often sources of hidden calories. Opt for water, herbal teas, or other unsweetened drinks.

>> ACTION POINTS - PRIORITY 1 <<

Spot the empty calories: Now that you are reading nutrition labels, keep an eye out for foods with high calories but low nutritional value

As you get used to reading food labels, you will understand the relationship between calories and nutrition. If you spot items with high calorie counts but little in terms of vitamins, minerals, or other beneficial nutrients, you are almost certainly looking at those 'empty calories' mentioned. Prioritise foods that offer more than just energy, but that nourish your body too.

Balance intake with expenditure: As you plan your meals, think about your daily activities

Think of your body as a car and food as its fuel. On days when you are mostly at rest, it does not need as much fuel and on days when you are moving around or engaging in physical activities, your body will require more energy. Before eating, pause for a moment to reflect on your day's plans. If it is a quiet day ahead, maybe opt for a salad or a light, healthy snack - but if you are expecting a busy or active day, go for an appropriately sized meal that will sustain you.

Mindful serving selection: Begin with a conscious glance at the 'serving size' on food labels during your next shopping trip

When you are next shopping and you are about to drop that packet into your basket, pause for a moment and take a quick look at the 'serving size' on the label. Remember, the serving size is just a guideline set by the manufacturer. Think about how much you would typically eat compared to what the food company believes to be 'a portion'.

Drink smart: When grabbing a drink, especially from cafes or coffee shops, be wary of those hidden calories

Next time you are tempted by a creamy latte or a sugary iced tea, just take a moment. Picture that drink alongside a meal, because in terms of calories, they might not be far apart. Instead of routinely picking up calorie-heavy options, why not choose plain water instead or consider herbal or green teas?

Food Labels - Fat

As we learnt earlier, not all fats are created equal. Some can be beneficial in moderation, while others might worsen health issues, complicate blood sugar control and compromise your heart health.

On food labels, 'fat' is listed as total fats and then are broken down further. Of course, 'total fats' are important to consider, as if nothing else they are very calorific when compared to carbohydrate and proteins. However, the breakdown of those fats is of particular importance to us.

Let us take a closer look at the food label:

- **Total fat:** This represents the total amount of all different fats in the product.
- **Saturated fats:** These are fats that are mainly from animal sources and are solid at room temperature.
- **Trans fats:** Typically resulting from a process that turns liquid fats into solids (hydrogenation), these are bad for your health.
- **Unsaturated fats:** These healthy fats are divided into monounsaturated and polyunsaturated, and are usually liquid at room temperature.
- **Omega-3 & Omega-6:** These are specific types of polyunsaturated fats and are especially beneficial for heart health.

While fats do not directly raise blood sugar, consuming too much can cause weight gain and impact insulin sensitivity. Choosing heart-healthy fats can help people with type 2 diabetes maintain balanced cholesterol levels and reduce the risk of heart-related problems. Including healthy fats in your diet can also curb overeating and the temptation to indulge in sugary snacks.

It is worth noting that not all might be as it seems on packaging and some food manufacturers may attempt to make their products seem healthier than they are.

Here are some of those claims to look out for:

- **"Low fat":** This does not mean 'healthy', as often when fat is reduced, sugar or artificial fillers can be added to compensate for flavour or texture.
- **"Fat-free":** Even if a product claims to be fat-free, it might be loaded with sugars.
- **"Made with healthy oils":** While the product might contain a healthy oil, it is important to check if it is the primary oil used, or if there are other less healthy fats present.

>> ACTION POINTS - PRIORITY 1 <<

Check the breakdown: Always look at the breakdown of fats
When you pick up a product, turn it around and look at the nutritional information. You will find a section detailing 'fats'. Look closely at the types of fats present - ideally, you want to see more of the unsaturated fats (like those found in olive oil or avocados) and less of the saturated and trans fats (often in processed foods and animal-based products). By making this simple yet effective habit, you are choosing heart-healthier options.

Serving size: Ensure you are clear on the serving size
Making foods seem healthier than they really are is a common trick played by the food industry. So, when you are out shopping, before being swayed by "low-fat" claims, always check the serving size indicated on the label. Ask yourself if it is a realistic portion for you. As an example, if a tin of soup claims to be low in fat per serving, but the tin contains two servings, you will consume twice the fat stated on the label if you eat the whole thing.

Limit saturated fats: Choose lean meats, use olive oil for cooking
When shopping for meat, look for labels showing 'lean' cuts or trim visible fats from your selection. When you are in the cooking oil aisle, reach for a bottle of olive oil which can be used for most culinary needs. By making minor tweaks, you are not just limiting saturated fats, but you are also introducing beneficial ones into your diet.

Avoid trans fats at all costs

Steering clear of trans fats can make a big difference to your health. When you are next shopping, take a moment to glance at the ingredients of packaged foods and keep an eye out for the term "partially hydrogenated oils". Seeing this is a telltale sign that trans fats are hidden inside.

>> ACTION POINT - PRIORITY 2 <<

Prioritise Omega-3s: Oily fish, walnuts and flaxseeds are excellent sources of Omega-3 fats

Next time you shop, add a tin of mackerel, a bag of walnuts, or a packet of flaxseeds to your basket. You can sprinkle flaxseeds on your morning steel-cut oats or Greek yoghurt, snack on a handful of walnuts, or enjoy a mackerel salad for lunch. By making these small additions to your meals, you will enrich your diet with heart-healthy fats.

Food Labels - Carbohydrates

We have established that carbohydrates have a direct influence on blood sugar levels, and that makes understanding the 'carbohydrates' data on food labels even more important.

Total carbohydrates

The 'total carbohydrates' figure on a food label represents all the carbohydrates in that product - inclusive of sugars, starches, and dietary fibres. Recognising this number can help gauge the potential impact a food item may have on your blood sugar levels (refer back to the sections on 'carbohydrate counting' and 'glycaemic index and load').

Dietary fibre

Listed under total carbohydrates, dietary fibre does not significantly raise blood sugar. In fact, high-fibre foods can assist in blood sugar management, making differentiating between total carbohydrate and dietary fibre a useful exercise.

Sugars

This subcategory shows the amount of naturally occurring and added sugars that are in the product. As it is these sugars that lead to swift spikes in blood glucose, these are of particular interest.

Sugar alcohols and net carbohydrates

On some labels, especially those on 'low-carbohydrate' products, you might see a mention of 'sugar alcohols'. They impact blood sugar less dramatically than regular sugars, but do still need to be accounted for. Some people subtract these and the dietary fibre from total carbs to get 'net carbs', which can be useful.

Before analysing carbohydrate content, ensure you are clear on the serving size. This helps in establishing the real impact of the food product on your daily carbohydrate intake. There may be more than one 'serving' in the box or packet. Some products might advertise as 'low-carb' by highlighting only net carbohydrates. Be sure to review the total carbohydrates and their constituents, like sugar alcohols, to assess their potential impact on your blood sugar levels.

Fresh fruits and vegetables rarely come with labels - they have no need to! When in doubt, opt for whole, unprocessed foods as they typically have a lower glycaemic index and are often higher in nutrients.

>> ACTION POINTS - PRIORITY 1 <<

Become a 'carb detective': Next time you are at the shops, take a moment to examine the 'total carbohydrates' on a few food labels

While shopping, pick up a few items and scan the 'total carbohydrates' section on their labels. Look for the breakdown of sugars, starches and dietary fibres. By understanding these elements, you will gain insight into how they might affect your blood sugar.

Embrace fibre-rich choices: Try incorporating more high-fibre foods into your meals
Start by incorporating whole foods into your meals - think whole grains like quinoa or barley, fresh fruits such as berries and leafy greens. When shopping, check food labels to see the dietary fibre content and aim for products higher in fibre. Over time, you will notice these wholesome additions not only keep your hunger at bay, but also help in maintaining stable blood sugar levels.

Natural over packaged: When in doubt, lean towards natural foods.
On your next shopping trip, dedicate more time to the fresh produce section and prioritise buying a variety of colourful fruits and veggies, aiming for what is in season. At home, keep them in sight – maybe in a fruit bowl on the counter or at eye level in the fridge. When you're hungry, these natural and nutritious options will be close by, making it simple to choose them over processed alternatives.

>> ACTION POINT - PRIORITY 2 <<

Stay serving-savvy: Before adding any item to your plate, double-check the serving size on its label
To become serving-savvy, always take a moment to scan the food label before eating. Notice the specified serving size and compare it to what you would usually consume. It is not just about the headline 'low-carb'

claim; dig deeper to check the full carbohydrate breakdown, including any hidden sugar alcohols. By making this a routine, you will ensure that what you consume aligns with your health goals and does not catch you off guard.

Food Labels - Sugars

'Sugars' on food labels can mean simple carbohydrates that are naturally occurring (like in fruits or milk) or added (like in biscuits, chocolates, and most processed foods). As most simple sugars quickly raise blood glucose levels and excessive consumption is closely linked with weight gain, being able to identify 'sugars' on food labels is essential.

'Total sugars': Most labels list 'total sugars', and these include both natural and added sugars, and it is important to differentiate between the two - naturally occurring sugars in fruits or dairy often come with beneficial nutrients, while added and refined sugars in processed foods do not.

Identifying 'added sugars': Some food labels might specify 'added sugars', which identifies sugars that are added during processing. If the label does not specify 'added sugars' then check the ingredients list for words like 'syrup', 'nectar', 'cane juice', or anything ending in '-ose' (like 'fructose' or 'dextrose'), as these all indicate added sugars.

Measurement units: On most food labels, sugars are listed in grams (g), and 4g of sugar is equivalent to about one teaspoon.

Deciphering sugar-related claims
- 'No added sugars' or 'unsweetened': products bearing these labels do not have any sugars added during processing, but that does not mean that they are sugar-free or indeed low in sugar. Check the label.
- 'Low sugar': for a product in the UK to be termed 'low sugar', it must contain no more than 5g of total sugars per 100g (or 2.5g of total sugars per 100ml for liquids).
- 'Sugar-free': this claim means the product contains less than 0.5g of sugar per serving, however it is crucial to check the serving size - as sometimes these can be unrealistically small, and you could easily eat or drink multiple servings in one sitting.

Hidden sugars and their impact

Sugar can masquerade under various names on ingredient lists, as we covered previously. Watch out for terms like 'honey', 'molasses', 'agave nectar', 'barley malt' and dozens more (they are all listed on my handy sugar-name pocket guide that I have put together for you).

'Sugar-free' or 'diet' products may contain artificial sweeteners like aspartame, saccharin, and steviol glycosides. While they offer sweetness without the calories, it's important to use them in moderation and consider their effect on your blood sugar levels.

Remember, natural sugars and added/refined sugars are not the same. While fruits contain natural sugars, they also offer fibre, vitamins and essential nutrients. Processed foods with added sugars often lack these benefits. Understanding the difference is key.

Please download my handy "sugar names" pocket guide, at www.diabetessolutions.co.uk/tkp-bonuspack

>> ACTION POINTS - PRIORITY 1 <<

Differentiate between natural and added sugars: While the term 'sugars' on food labels encompasses various simple carbohydrates, it is important to determine the source

To easily differentiate sugars, start by scanning the ingredients on food labels. Ingredients are listed by quantity, so if sugar-related terms appear at the beginning (or in the first half of the ingredients list), that is a clue. Keep an eye out for words ending in '-ose' (like 'fructose') and others such as 'syrup'. These often indicate added sugars.

Be wary of sugar-related claims: Claims like 'no added sugars', 'low sugar' and 'sugar-free' sound promising but require a closer look

Do not take sugar-related claims at face value - a label boasting 'no added sugars' might still have high natural sugars. For 'low sugar' claims, quickly check the nutritional information: it should be up to 5g per 100g or 2.5g per 100ml for drinks. For 'sugar-free' products, scrutinise the serving size, ensuring it is a realistic amount for you (and check to see that it is not packed with artificial sweeteners).

Embrace whole foods: The old adage "nature knows best" rings especially true here

When shopping, consider heading to the fresh produce aisle first. Here, you will find the most nutritious foods in the shop. Fruit offers fibre and essential nutrients that benefit your blood sugar balance. Start with minor changes: if you fancy a sweet treat, try swapping that biscuit for an apple. Over time, this habit will not only satiate your sugar cravings but also provide your body with nourishing goodness.

Food Labels - Sodium

Sodium is essential for maintaining fluid balance, muscle function, and nerve transmission in our body.

It is typically listed in milligrams (mg) per serving and keep in mind that your primary concern should be your 'salt' intake. To determine the 'salt' content from the sodium amount, multiply the sodium amount by 2.5.

The recommended salt intake for adults is no more than 6g per day (equivalent to about 2.4g of sodium). Keep this figure in mind when assessing products.

Evaluating sodium claims on labels
- 'Low sodium': For a product to be considered 'low sodium' in the UK, it must contain no more than 0.12g of sodium (or 0.3g of salt) per 100g or 100ml.
- 'Very low sodium': Products with this claim should have no more than 0.04g of sodium (or 0.1g of salt) per 100g or 100ml.
- 'Reduced sodium': This indicates the product contains at least 25% less sodium than the regular version. However, it does not mean the product is low in sodium.

\>\> ACTION POINTS - PRIORITY 1 \<\<

Understand the difference between salt and sodium: While sodium is a component of salt, they are not the same

To understand the salt content in foods, always check the 'sodium' figure on the label - and then multiply this number by 2.5 to get the equivalent salt amount. For instance, if a product contains 2g of sodium per serving, that is 5g of salt. By making this quick calculation, you will get a clearer picture of your salt intake.

Monitor your daily intake: Aim for the recommended limit of no more than 6g of salt (or roughly 2.4g of sodium) per day

Start by setting a daily goal, like the 2.4g sodium recommendation. When you are shopping, scan product labels for the sodium content. Perhaps even use a food diary app to keep track. By noting these figures, you will be more aware of how close you are to your limit.

Be a savvy shopper: When you are looking at food labels, be vigilant about spotting ingredients that signal higher sodium content

Next time you shop, take a quick look at the ingredients list for sodium clues like 'monosodium glutamate' or 'sodium bicarbonate'. These are indicators of higher sodium content. In addition, do not be swayed by 'reduced sodium' or 'reduced salt' claims and instead, compare it to the regular version to see how much difference there really is.

\>\> ACTION POINT - PRIORITY 2 <<

Prioritise balance in your diet: Remember, it is all about striking a balance

Start by looking at food labels for sodium content when shopping. Choose fresh over processed foods, when possible, as they naturally contain less sodium. If you fancy a meal that is high in sodium, pair it with lower sodium choices for the day to strike that balance.

Food Labels - Fibre

We often see 'total fibre' or 'total dietary fibre' on a food label, and it denotes the combined amount of both soluble and insoluble fibre together. As foods with fibre in them often contain both types, they are rarely (if ever) separated on a food label.

In relation to blood sugar control, fibre content should not be viewed in isolation, as it is often listed under the broader 'carbohydrates' category. Therefore, it is important to compare the fibre content against the total carbohydrates, especially when looking for foods that may have a lower impact on blood sugar levels. The higher the fibre-to-carbohydrate ratio, the better.

Decoding food label claims

- 'High in fibre': labels might state that a product is 'high in fibre'. In the UK, for a product to make this claim, it should contain at least 6g of fibre per 100g.
- 'Source of fibre': indicates that the product contains at least 3g of fibre per 100g.

Reaching 25-30g per day of fibre can help control blood sugar levels and bring other health benefits like reducing cancer risk and improving gut health. Fibre-rich foods also are more filling, helping to reduce overall food intake and therefore assisting with weight management.

Natural sources of fibre are best as, while 'fortified' foods can offer added fibre, natural sources like fruits, vegetables, legumes and whole grains are often richer in nutrients and provide a balanced intake of both soluble and insoluble fibres. In addition, some so-called high-fibre processed foods (like cereals) may also be high in added sugars. Always balance the fibre content against the sugar content, ensuring you are not inadvertently increasing your sugar intake in your efforts to consume more fibre.

>> ACTION POINTS - PRIORITY 1 <<

Prioritise the 'total dietary fibre' on labels
Locate the 'total dietary fibre' on food labels - this number is a mix of both vital fibre types and is a handy guide to gauge a product's goodness. Remember that soluble fibre is great for balancing blood sugar and cholesterol, and insoluble fibre keeps your digestion moving smoothly.

Balance fibre with overall carbohydrates
When shopping, make it a habit to first glance at the 'total carbohydrates' on food labels and then immediately check the 'dietary fibre' beneath it. Aim for foods where the fibre forms a good portion of those carbohydrates. For example, a food item that has 20g of total carbohydrates and 5g of fibre is a good balance. By choosing foods with a higher fibre-to-carbohydrate ratio, you are going some way to controlling your blood sugar levels.

>> ACTION POINTS - PRIORITY 2 <<

Spotting 'high in fibre' or 'source of fibre' on a product might feel like a win, but make sure it genuinely is!

When food manufacturers make a big thing on packaging about their product being 'high in fibre' or a 'source of fibre', do not just take their word for it. Quickly check the label: is there 6g of fibre per 100g for the former and 3g for the latter? Good - now glance at the 'total carbohydrates'. How does the fibre measure up? For better blood sugar control, look for foods where the fibre makes up a good chunk of those carbohydrates.

Choose natural, but stay alert: There's nothing quite like natural sources of fibre

When you are shopping, naturally fibre-rich foods like fruits and vegetables are a superb choice. If you are drawn to a packaged 'high-fibre' product then scan the label for added sugars. Even if it is rich in fibre, excessive sugar can counteract those benefits. Always weigh the fibre against the sugar content and let this balance guide your decision.

Food Labels - Protein

The amount of protein in a product is typically listed in grams (g) per serving, and you would do well to compare this with your recommended daily intake (as a guide 0.75g per kg of body weight for the average person, increasing to 1-1.25g per kg for a very active person, although this amount may vary from individual to individual, so please consult a suitable health professional for your specific amount).

Not all proteins are created equal, as the source and type of protein can vary in their amino acid profiles. Animal sources are often 'complete proteins', meaning they provide all essential amino acids. Plant-based proteins can be 'incomplete', requiring combinations to ensure all amino acids are present. The ingredients list can give clues about where the protein comes from, such as soy, lentils, milk, chicken, or fish.

Protein claims on food labels
- 'High protein': In the UK, for food to be labelled 'high protein', at least 20% of its energy value should be provided by protein.
- 'Source of protein': This label means the product provides at least 12% of its energy value from protein. Again, it is always good to check the total grams of protein per serving.

- For plant-based products, you might encounter labels like 'combined proteins' or 'complementary proteins'. These indicate that the product combines different plant sources to offer a complete protein profile.

>> ACTION POINTS - PRIORITY 1 <<

Always check the protein amount: When shopping, take a moment to glance at the protein content mentioned in grams per serving on the food label
Develop the habit of quickly checking the protein content on food labels and familiarise yourself with your personal daily protein needs. With this knowledge in hand, when you see the grams of protein per serving, you can easily assess if a product aligns with your dietary goals.

Understand the source: Remember, not all proteins are the same
Look at the ingredients list and identify protein sources like soy, lentils, or meats such as chicken. This will help you balance the amino acids you consume.

>> ACTION POINTS - PRIORITY 2 <<

Decode protein claims: Be savvy about labels
Give those 'high protein' and 'source of protein' labels a second glance and understand their real meaning. When you spot 'high protein', it

signifies a significant percentage of its calories come from protein. If it says 'source of protein', it is still a reasonable amount but less.

Celebrate plant-based combinations: If you are venturing into plant-based options, keep an eye out for labels mentioning 'combined proteins' or 'complementary proteins'

When embracing plant-based diets, look out for labels like 'combined proteins' or 'complementary proteins'. These labels mean the product brings together various plant sources to give you all the essential amino acids you need.

Food Labels - Vitamins and Minerals

When looking at food labels, we often focus attention on the macronutrients, the numbers, the percentages, and the ingredients. However, it is also worth looking at the vitamin and mineral content too, as some of these can positively influence blood sugar control.

Vitamins (organic compounds needed in small amounts) play a role in growth, digestion, nerve function and other processes. Minerals (inorganic compounds that are found in soil or water) are important for bone health, heart health, and cognitive function.

Like many other countries, the UK doesn't require food manufacturers to list every vitamin and mineral in a product, only the important ones or those being promoted on the packaging. Commonly, you will find vitamin D, calcium, and iron on food labels, but others might be listed if they are fortified in the product or if the product naturally has a significant amount.

When looking at a food label, the %DV (daily value) or %RI (reference intake) tells you the percentage of each nutrient in a single serving, in relation to the daily recommended amount for the 'average person'. If the %DV (or %RI) is 15%, that means the food provides 15% of the average person's daily needs for that nutrient, per serving.

Key vitamins and minerals for type 2 diabetes

- Magnesium: Magnesium deficiency can affect the function of insulin.
- Vitamin D: Low vitamin D levels have been linked to insulin resistance.
- Chromium: There's some evidence that chromium might help to regulate blood sugar.

Evaluating claims on labels

Be wary of labels making grand claims about vitamin and mineral content. Phrases like "packed with essential vitamins" or "rich in minerals" can be misleading. Always turn to the nutritional information to see the exact amounts and %DV (%RI).

It is best to get your vitamins and minerals from natural food sources; but supplements can be useful in some situations and should only be considered under guidance. While some vitamins and minerals can be beneficial, over-consumption is not recommended as excessive intake of some vitamins and minerals can be harmful.

>> ACTION POINT - PRIORITY 1 <<

Prioritise whole foods

Whenever you shop, fill your basket predominantly with whole foods like fresh fruits, leafy greens, nuts, and whole grains. These are full of the vitamins and minerals that our bodies need.

>> ACTION POINTS - PRIORITY 2 <<

Embrace fortified foods mindfully

Fortified foods can be a wise choice for the nutrients that you are lacking in. As you pick up that fortified cereal or plant-based drink, take a quick moment to scan the label. While the added vitamins and minerals are great, do not let hidden sugars sneak past your radar. It is about finding that balance: embracing the nutrient boost while sidestepping unnecessary extras.

Seek guidance before diving deep: While I am all for empowering you to make informed choices, there is no harm in seeking a bit of expert advice now and then

Before making big changes or adding supplements, consider scheduling a chat with a nutrition expert. They are a treasure trove of tailored advice and, remember, asking for a little guidance is both wise and proactive.

The Traffic Light Food Label System

The traffic light food label system was designed to speed up your ability to get a good idea of how healthy (or unhealthy) a particular food or drink is at a glance. Nutrients commonly displayed on the label are fats, saturated fats, sugars, and salt. It can be a useful tool, but needs to be understood and used properly.

Each 1/2 pack serving (150g) contains:

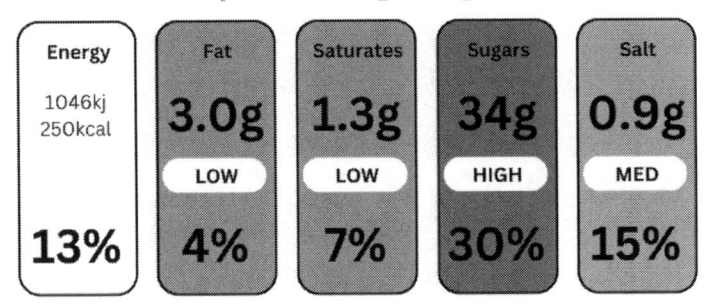

Energy	Fat	Saturates	Sugars	Salt
1046kj 250kcal	3.0g LOW	1.3g LOW	34g HIGH	0.9g MED
13%	4%	7%	30%	15%

of an adult's reference intake.
Typical values (as sold) per 100g: 697kj / 167kcal

This system uses three colours to indicate the level of specific nutrients in a product:

- Green indicates a low amount.
- Amber signals a medium amount.
- Red warns of a high amount.

With a quick look, you can gauge the nutritional profile of a product and compare it to other products. You can also quickly identify those with lower sugars or fats, helping maintain stable blood glucose levels.

The system seems perfect, almost too good to be true - especially for those who have trouble understanding the nutritional information on packaging.

And yes, sadly, it is too good to be true. Not that it is an inherently bad system by any means, but you need to balance the colours you see on the label with some background knowledge - specifically of how some food companies can manipulate the data, and of how you can be subconsciously influenced by the colours you see.

Over-reliance on colour

Let us assume for a moment that a product is showing green for fats, saturates and sat, but red for sugars. You might be drawn to the green and inadvertently ignore the red. But just because fats are green and sugars are red does not automatically qualify it as being a 'healthy' or 'unhealthy' option. Decisions should be balanced, considering the complete nutritional makeup, not just one factor or colour.

Manipulating serving sizes

Some manufacturers might adjust serving sizes down as small as possible to manipulate the figures, ensuring they land in the 'green' zone and therefore they can make their product look healthier than it really is. Because these tiny serving sizes are not representative of a realistic serving size, you might consume double or triple that amount, leading to an unintended calorie/salt/sugar/fat overload.

Neglect of other nutrients

The traffic light system is focused is predominantly on fats, sugars and salt - and leaves out the other nutrients like fibre, protein, or specific vitamins. The traffic light system rarely includes "total carbohydrates". When trying to control blood sugar levels, it is important to monitor total carbohydrates, so check the detailed information on the back.

Natural vs added sugars

The traffic light system does not differentiate between naturally occurring sugars (like those found in fruits) and added, refined and processed sugars. This can be misleading, especially when comparing fruit-based products to processed or artificially sweetened ones.

The 'healthy' halo effect

It is easy to be misled into thinking that just because a product boasts mostly green labels, it must be 'healthy'. Other ingredients, additives, or chemical preservatives not considered in the colours, and it can be these that negatively impact your health and blood glucose levels.

>> ACTION POINTS - PRIORITY 1 <<

Interpret with balance: When glancing at those traffic light labels, do not get swayed by a single green
Let the traffic light labels be your guide, but not the final verdict. While a green for sugars is enticing, take a moment to see what the fats say. Be sure to look beyond a single colour and seek a blend of green and the occasional amber to ensure you are making smart choices.

Distinguish sugars: The traffic light does not tell tales of sugar origin
If a product claims to be 'fruit-sweetened', check the ingredients list to confirm. If you see terms like 'fruit concentrate' or the name of a fruit itself, that is a nod towards natural sugars. Words like 'glucose syrup' or 'fructose' are clues to added and unhealthy sugars. Over time, this little extra effort helps you differentiate the wholesome choices from the more processed options.

Realistic servings matter: Some labels look friendly because of tiny serving sizes
Give the serving size on labels a closer look and ask yourself, "does it match what I would typically eat?". If not, attempt to make mental adjustments to the colours of those traffic lights. For example, a small bowl of cereal might be marked as 'one serving', but if you usually have a larger bowl, those nutrient amounts will increase. It is all about being mindful and realistic about your portions.

>> ACTION POINTS - PRIORITY 2 <<

Look beyond the big three: While fats, sugars and salt are highlighted, remember they are not the entire story

Take a moment to delve deeper than those traffic light labels. Turn the product over and familiarise yourself with the finer details on the nutritional information label and ingredients list. The detailed nutritional breakdown provides a complete picture, while the colourful indicators on the front give only a summary. In the context of blood sugar control, spotting 'total carbohydrates' is essential.

Avoid the 'healthy halo' trap: Just because a product has a number of 'greens', it does not automatically make it healthy

When you spot a product boasting all green labels, it is natural to think that the product is healthy. Before adding it to your basket, check the ingredients list on the packaging for any unfamiliar or lengthy names that could indicate additives or preservatives. Opt for products with shorter, recognisable ingredient lists. By taking a moment to look beyond the traffic lights, you are choosing foods that truly support your health.

Type 2 Diabetes-Supporting Supplements

So far, we have covered some basics of nutrition, of how what you eat and drink can affect your blood sugar levels, and how these can affect your overall health.

I would now like to spend a moment looking at some supplements that can improve your blood sugar levels and, potentially, your wellbeing too.

You might wonder why I have included a section on supplements in my book? Well, whilst I am an advocate for a balanced, natural, whole foods diet (and believe it is the cornerstone of good health), I also appreciate that modern-day problems such as soil depletion, industrialised farming and dietary changes have led to decreased nutrient content in even whole foods.

I will not go into great detail about each supplement, but I hope this section sparks some interest in you to research further. As a rule of thumb, when it comes to any supplementation, you should buy the most expensive that you can afford, as not all supplements are created equal.

Disclaimer: Before we continue, I must temper the subject of supplementation for blood sugar control with caution.

While the supplements discussed in this section have shown some promise in supporting blood sugar control, they should NOT be considered a replacement for medication and if you are on medication for type 2 diabetes, be cautious. Be cautious about taking natural supplements with your medication as they may lower your blood sugar too much.

I have intentionally omitted serving sizes or doses of these supplements, as they will vary depending on your personal situation and any supplementation should be seen as part of a broader strategy, inclusive of diet, exercise, and regular medical checks.

It is important to check with your doctor first to see if these supplements are safe for you, especially if you are taking other medication.

Berberine

Berberine, found in a variety of plants (including the Barberry, Goldenseal and Oregon grape) has been used in traditional Chinese medicine for centuries, and has become more widely known in recent years for its medicinal properties in relation to blood glucose control.

It has been called "Nature's Metformin" and for good reason, as Berberine has been observed to behave similar to insulin in its ability to transport glucose into cells - which may help cells to become more receptive to insulin. It could also help to inhibit glucose production of the liver, which helps in blood sugar control.

Gymnema Sylvestre

Gymnema Sylvestre is a climbing shrub native to India, Africa, and Australia. Its leaves are used in Ayurvedic medicine for controlling blood sugar levels.

The compounds in it can control blood sugar levels by blocking sugar receptors in the intestines, reducing sugar absorption and promoting insulin release. It may also enhance pancreatic beta cell growth.

Interestingly, the Hindi name for Gymnema Sylvestre is 'Gurmar', which translates to 'sugar destroyer'.

Astaxanthin

Astaxanthin (pronounced as-ta-zan-thin) is a powerful antioxidant and anti-inflammatory compound. Carotenoids are natural pigments made by plants and algae to protect themselves. When we consume carotenoids, they can also protect our cells from oxidative stress.

Oxidative stress plays a role in type 2 diabetes, and by its function as an antioxidant in neutralising free radicals, Astaxanthin may protect the cells of the pancreas. By decreasing triglycerides and boosting HDL cholesterol, it might improve lipid profiles.

The most natural dietary source of Astaxanthin is wild-caught salmon. Supplementation is often preferred because of the need for higher concentrations to experience therapeutic benefits. If you consider supplementation, ensure that it is sourced from natural marine algae rather than synthetically produced.

Moringa

Moringa, known as the 'drumstick tree' or 'miracle tree,' comes from the sub-Himalayan regions of India, Pakistan, and Afghanistan and has gained attention for its health benefits. In addition to vitamins C, A, and E, moringa leaves contain calcium, potassium, and iron. These leaves are also rich in antioxidants that help manage blood sugar levels, combat oxidative stress, reduce inflammation and has also shown potential in aiding the reduction of cholesterol levels.

Chia Seeds

Chia seeds, once used by the ancient Mayan and Aztec cultures for their energy-boosting properties, come from the Salvia Hispanica plant. They are small, oval-shaped seeds that can absorb large amounts of water, expanding up to 10-12 times their size when soaked.

Chia seeds are high in fibre, high in Omega-3 fatty acids, protein, calcium, and antioxidants. Being high in fibre, chia seeds can slow down the rate at which food is digested and sugar is released into the bloodstream, which helps to reduce sudden spikes in blood sugar after eating.

By improving blood sugar responses after meals, chia seeds can, over time, help the body respond better to insulin too.

Vitamin D

Vitamin D is a fat-soluble vitamin that we primarily gain from sunlight exposure, though it can also be found in certain foods and supplements too. We associate it with calcium and good bone health, but vitamin D is also linked to improved metabolic health.

Vitamin D has been shown to improve sensitivity as well as promoting good pancreatic health. It is also an effective anti-inflammatory as well as playing an important role in maintaining calcium balance in the body (there is a close relationship between calcium metabolism, and insulin secretion and utilisation).

With the increasing prevalence of more sedentary lifestyles, working from home and sunscreen usage, Vitamin D deficiency has become more of an issue in recent years.

Aloe Vera

Aloe Vera is a succulent plant from the Arabian peninsula. It has thick leaves filled with a gel-like substance. It is well-known for its use on burns and skin irritations. Aloe Vera has some interesting internal benefits too, particularly in relation to the control of blood sugars.

Consumption of Aloe Vera may help to enhance the body's insulin response, making it more efficient in transporting glucose from the bloodstream into cells and the compounds in Aloe Vera have been shown to have anti-glycaemic effects, so they could help in lowering post-meal blood glucose levels.

Aloe Vera contains antioxidants and enzymes that may reduce inflammation, a factor in insulin resistance.

Cinnamon

The compounds in cinnamon have anti-inflammatory and antioxidant effects, mimic insulin, and slow down digestion to control blood sugar levels.

By inhibiting certain digestive enzymes, Cinnamon also slows down the metabolism of carbohydrates in the digestive tract, so the glucose is released into the bloodstream at a steadier, more manageable rate.

There are two primary types of cinnamon – Ceylon and cassia. Cassia is more commonly found in supermarkets, but it contains higher levels of coumarin, a natural compound that can be harmful in large doses. For regular consumption, especially for health reasons, Ceylon cinnamon is the safer choice. It is sometimes referred to as "true" cinnamon and has a subtler, sweeter flavour.

Magnesium

Magnesium plays an important role in your health, helping your muscles and nerves to function properly. Around 60% of the magnesium in your body is found in your bones, with the rest in your muscles, soft tissue and fluids. Magnesium is important for how the body responds to insulin, and not having enough can make insulin less effective.

Sadly today, magnesium deficiency is quite common as modern agricultural practices (including overworking the ground) often strip essential minerals from the soil, which reduces the nutrient content of foods grown in that soil. To compound the problem, today many people have diets are dominated by processed foods, and these are low in magnesium.

If you are looking to improve your magnesium levels (please check your levels first, certainly before supplementing), you could integrate more magnesium-rich foods in your diet including leafy green vegetables (e.g., spinach), nuts (especially almonds and cashews), seeds (like chia and flaxseeds), whole grains and legumes. If you don't get enough magnesium from your diet or need more, magnesium supplements can help.

There are different types of magnesium supplement, and each serve a different purpose - so it's important to take them with guidance.

Remember, whilst it is important to keep your magnesium levels up by consuming whole foods (or supplementing where appropriate), you need to consider existing dietary factors that might hinder its absorption - like issues with your gut health and other components of your diet (for example, excessive alcohol and caffeine intake can hinder magnesium absorption).

Chromium

Chromium is a trace mineral, and it plays an important part in your general health and in your ability to control blood sugar levels. Though required in tiny amounts, chromium plays several important roles in your body, including assisting in the metabolism of carbohydrates, fats and proteins, helping to improve the function of insulin and also reducing insulin resistance.

Good sources of chromium include nuts, whole grains, lean meats, fruits, and vegetables like broccoli, oranges, and green beans.

My Two Golden Rules

— The '10,000 year' rule —

In the rapidly evolving world of today, where technology influences almost every facet of our lives and unhealthy, processed food is readily available, one thing remains relatively unchanged - our human physiology.

Despite significant changes in our surroundings and cultures, our bodies have remained relatively unchanged for the past 10,000 years.

Our ancestors thrived on fruit and vegetables that they cultivated, the animals they hunted, the fish they caught and the edibles like nuts, seeds and berries that they foraged. These foods, unaltered and unprocessed, nourished their bodies, providing them with the necessary nutrients.

However, as humans transitioned from a hunter-gatherer society to an industrialised one, our diets underwent dramatic changes and today food has become more about convenience and shelf life - which heralded the introduction of processed and ultra-processed foods into our diets. These foods often have crucial nutrients stripped away and harmful additives included, creating the nutritional paradox of calorie-rich but nutrient-poor food.

Put simply, today most people fuel their bodies with food created by companies who are very unlikely to have our best interests (or health!) at heart. We are not designed to run efficiently on such 'junk' processed and ultra-processed foods.

The consequences of ignoring our roots

Our modern diets, dominated by sugars, unhealthy fats and synthetic additives, are at odds with the diet that our bodies thrive on - and this mismatch can often lead to health issues including nutritional deficiencies (where essential nutrients found abundantly in whole foods are simply not present in processed and ultra-processed foods), metabolic disorders (an over-reliance on sugars and unhealthy fats that can lead to diseases like type 2 diabetes) and gut issues (where a lack of dietary fibre and the presence of additives can disrupt our gut's microbiome, leading on to other health problems).

Embracing the 10,000 year rule

If our bodies haven't changed much over 10,000 years, then perhaps we need to make sure that our diets should not either - and make a conscious effort to eat whole, natural foods when we can.

You can integrate my 10,000-year rule to your daily diet by prioritising whole foods first - fruits, vegetables, lean meats, fish, nuts and seeds. These foods are dense in nutrients and devoid of harmful additives. If a food item is processed or ultra-processed, comes a tin or a packet or has a long ingredient list full of terms you cannot pronounce, then reconsider its place in your diet.

When you are making your food (and drink) choices, stop for a moment and ask yourself: "Might I have been able to get this 10,000 years ago"? If the answer is no, choose something that is.

By adopting my 10,000-year rule, you are embracing a dietary philosophy tailored to your biological needs as a human being. It is a step back in time to propel your health forward. Day to day and particularly when the next time you find yourself in the grocery aisle or at a restaurant, please consider this principle - as it will help you make smarter dietary choices.

Similar to my '10,000 year' golden rule, but unique in its own way, the 'catch it, grow it, rear it' principle is another easy-to-follow guide to help you make better food choices.

— The 'catch it, grow it, rear it' rule —

In a world overwhelmed with diet fads, processed foods and conflicting nutritional advice, it is easy to feel lost when it comes to making the right food choices. Amid this dietary confusion, simplicity can often be the most effective.

This leads us to my second golden rule: "can you catch it, can you grow it or can you rear it?". At its core, the principle is a guide for determining the naturalness and wholesomeness of your food choices.

When you are about to eat, pause and ask yourself:

- Could I catch this.
- Or could I grow it.
- Or could I rear it.

If the answer to any of these questions is "yes", you are likely on the right track. If it is "no", it is time for some dietary introspection and different choices.

Why these rules matter

This rule encourages you to consume foods that are closer to their natural state, nourishing your body the way nature intended. Foods that fit the "catch it, grow it, rear it" rule are typically free from harmful additives, preservatives, artificial ingredients and are minimally processed, ensuring you get pure nutritional value.

In our modern age of convenience, we often sacrifice quality for ease. My "10,000 year" and "catch it, grow it, rear it" golden rules offers simple approach to making healthier food choices and can be used by anyone, anywhere and at any time.

Step 1 Summary

As step 1 draws to a close, please do reflect on the nutrition knowledge that you have gained so far, as it will help to guide your food and drink decisions now and (if you allow it) for the rest of your life. Where you feel you need to, please do go back over the topics as needed, and do more research if you want to.

I hope that you have lots of positive 'Action Points' to begin working on, starting today. Some of these points you will no doubt put in to place straight away (especially the "Must Do's") and they will begin to make an immediate difference in your life; others might take a little longer to show any tangible results - but please stay committed to these changes and do not give up.

Focus on being better today than you were yesterday and better tomorrow than you are today. This is not a sprint; this is a marathon. Pace yourself. Be kind to yourself and remember that every step in the right direction is - no matter how small - a step in the right direction.

As I mentioned earlier, your journey is unique to you, so take it as fast or as slow as you are comfortable with to make it work for you. Make the process fluid, and adjust and add to it as you need to, and as you go along.

Remember that the philosophy underpinning my KISSS Plan is about progress and not perfection. Allow yourself the latitude to make mistakes, to mess things up, to not get things right all the time. That is perfectly okay.

I hope that the information and action points I have given to you all make sense. If not, or you are struggling to find ways to put what you have learnt in to practise, then do book a free 15 minute Zoom or phone session with me at **www.diabetessolutions.co.uk/support-sessions** and I will be happy to help you.

I am now going to build on step 1 and take you through step 2 - and encourage you to move more (particularly if you have quite a sedentary lifestyle).

Step 2: Get Moving!

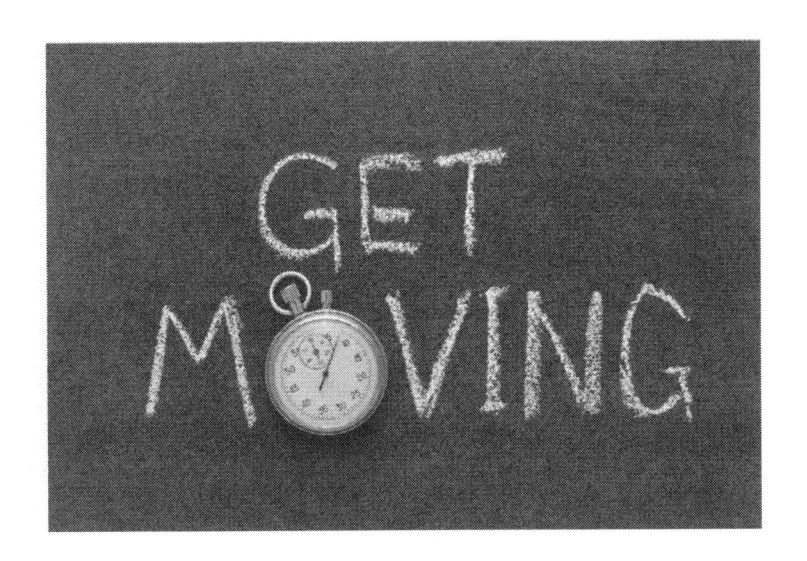

Introduction

Welcome to Step 2 – Movement

Engaging in regular physical activity is undeniably beneficial. However, the very mention of 'exercise' often conjures up images of packed gyms, heavy weights and rigorous training schedules - and if you enjoy that sort of thing, then I applaud you.

For the rest of us to who would prefer to stay away from a gym, there are still many exercises that you can do at home, often for little cost.

Remember what we learnt in step 1 - one of the root causes of type 2 diabetes is the body's inability to make use of insulin properly, which leads to sustained elevated blood sugar levels. Regular movement (note, 'movement', not necessarily 'exercise') has been shown to help insulin work more efficiently, even if weight loss (if you are trying to lose weight) is not immediately evident. Movement (and, of course, by extension, exercise) can lead to improved blood sugar control, increased insulin sensitivity and the prospect of preventing type 2 diabetes in the first place or reversing it if you already have it.

When we talk about 'movement', it is important to understand it is a wide spectrum. From a gentle walk in the park or stretching exercises at your desk to more structured activities like yoga or swimming, it all counts. Every step taken and every lap around the block can take you closer to that goal of improved health.

Ultimately, what matters is that you find enjoyment in whatever activity you do and making movement a routine part of your daily life.

Make a promise to yourself right now to be more active if you lead a sedentary lifestyle. Your future self will appreciate it.

As in step 1, sections in step 2 have several 'priority 1 and 'priority 2 action points. Whilst reading through step 2, please note down on your 'Action Points worksheet' those that are relevant, beneficial, and that you will be working on.

Do not forget to download the bonus material at www.diabetessolutions.co.uk/tkp-bonuspack

(Note: I am not a personal trainer but fully advocate movement and exercise in preventing and reversing type 2 diabetes. Prior to embarking on any exercise routine (especially those that you are not used to or are unfamiliar with) I recommend consulting first with your doctor and/or a fitness professional).

Activity Boosts Energy Levels

Regular movement improves blood circulation and boosts energy levels. By expending energy through movement, you can actually gain more of it - and here is how:

At the heart of your body's energy production is a molecule called Adenosine Triphosphate (ATP). When you engage in any form of activity, your body breaks down ATP to release and use this energy. Your daily diet is the primary source from which this ATP is generated (which is another reason your dietary choices are important!) and as you move, your muscles demand more energy, which prompts an increase in the rate of ATP production.

With physical activity, your heart rate rises, and blood circulation improves. Enhanced blood circulation ensures that oxygen (a critical component in the energy production process) reaches your muscles efficiently. This facilitates the swift conversion of nutrients into energy.

Your cells contain tiny structures known as Mitochondria (often termed the 'powerhouses' of the cell) and engaging in consistent daily movement prompts the growth of more Mitochondria in your cells, leading to increased energy production. Regular movement helps maintain a steady energy supply by using glucose effectively, preventing fatigue from blood sugar fluctuations.

Beyond the cellular level, the link between movement and energy is deeply rooted in your mental wellbeing too, as physical activity prompts the release of endorphins, your body's natural mood elevators. Endorphins often lead to what is popularly known as the 'runner's high', but interestingly, it does not require intensive exercise to achieve. Even a brisk walk can trigger this uplifting sensation. Regular movement has also been shown to counter chronic fatigue more effectively than static rest and an active body often translates to better sleep. Quality sleep is crucial for energy restoration. Consistent movement can help regulate sleep patterns, ensuring we wake up refreshed and recharged.

>> ACTION POINTS - PRIORITY 1 <<

Start slowly: If you are new to incorporating regular physical activity, it is essential to start at a pace that feels comfortable

Choose shorter sessions initially, perhaps a 10-minute daily walk or light stretching exercises at home. As your stamina builds, gradually increase your activity duration or intensity. By following this approach, you can maintain your energy levels without draining them, allowing your body to adapt comfortably and sustainably. Remember, it is progress, not perfection, that counts.

Consistency is key: It is not about how much you do in a single day, but about creating a routine
Begin by allocating specific times for activity, even if it is just a brief walk after meals or a short morning stretch. As these small activities become a habit, they anchor your day, giving you predictable energy boosts. Over time, you will find that this rhythm not only elevates your energy, but also nurtures your overall wellbeing. Small, daily steps can create lasting, energetic changes in your life.

Listen to your body: On some days, you might feel more energetic than on others
If you wake up feeling vibrant and full of energy, perhaps it is a good day for a more intense workout. On quieter days, a gentle stroll or some light stretching might be best. Adjusting your activity level based on how you feel ensures you are nourishing your body without overtaxing it. Think of it as having a friendly chat with your body each day, asking "What shall we do today?" and then listening to its response.

>> ACTION POINT - PRIORITY 2 <<

Include variety: Different forms of movement offer varied benefits
Take a walk or a bike ride around your neighbourhood one day, and the next day, do some gentle weightlifting or resistance band exercises at home. Do not forget to sprinkle in some yoga or stretches to keep your muscles limber. By rotating your activities, you keep things fresh and engaging, and ensure a boost to your energy and wellbeing.

Activity Supports Mental Health

Living with type 2 diabetes can be challenging; from checking your blood sugars daily, to having to think about what you eat and drink, and then worrying over long-term issues. It can all become quite exhausting, leading to feeling of stress, anxiety and sometimes, even depression. These feelings can also have a negative effect on your blood sugar levels - creating a cycle that can be difficult to break.

But here is some good news - regular movement and activity (whether that might be a simple walk or a workout down the gym) helps your body to release endorphins. Endorphins are chemicals that act as painkillers and mood elevators, and which create feelings of happiness that can counteract anxiety or low mood.

Staying active helps your brain too by increasing blood flow and improving the delivery of oxygen and other nutrients. These nourish the brain and support the production of hormones that encourage the growth of brain cells - helping to sharpen cognitive function and memory over time, and potentially reducing the risk of cognitive decline and diseases like Alzheimer's in the longer term.

So, remember… regular activity and movement can go a long way in improving, not just your physical health, but your mental health too!

Incorporating Exercise Into Daily Activity

When you are active, your muscles make use of the glucose in your blood, which helps to control your blood sugar levels. Incorporating regular movement into your daily routine does not mean having to do strenuous workouts or going down to the gym. Being 'active' can be easier than you might think, as even a daily 10-minute jog or a 20-minute walk can be effective.

If you are not used to exercise, you may decide to start small and then gradually increase the duration and intensity as you gain confidence and stamina. Instead of setting vague objectives like "I will be more active", opt for SMART goals such as "I will walk for 20 minutes after dinner every day". When you are out and about, choose the stairs over the lift, park further from the entrance of shops, or do simple stretches while watching television.

The key to optimal exercise results is being consistent. It's better to walk for 20 minutes each day rather than doing one intense hour of exercise and then being inactive for weeks. Be sure to choose activities you enjoy and resonate with you - if you love nature, hiking might be your best bet. If music uplifts you, dancing might be the perfect choice.

>> ACTION POINTS - PRIORITY 1 <<

Start the day with movement: Whether it is a series of stretches or a brisk walk

To integrate activity into your morning routine, set aside just ten minutes after you wake up. This could be as simple as stretching your arms and legs in bed or taking a brisk walk around your garden or close neighbourhood. You do not need any specific equipment; just a commitment to start the day with movement.

Daily steps

Incorporating more steps into your day is an easy way to increase your activity, so begin by setting a daily goal, perhaps 5,000 steps if you are just starting out. Download a step-tracking app on to your phone (or use a pedometer) and throughout the day, look for small opportunities to walk: take the stairs, park further from the door when you go shopping, or enjoy a brisk walk during your lunch break. Over time, you will probably enjoy and find satisfaction from gradually increasing your step goal.

Stay hydrated

Make it a habit to carry a reusable water bottle with you throughout the day. Having it within reach will act as a gentle reminder to sip regularly. It is not just about quenching thirst, but ensuring your body operates optimally, especially when you are active.

Set clear goals: Having clear, measurable goals can be motivating
Start by deciding what you want to focus on: perhaps a daily step count of 5,000 steps or 30 minutes of brisk walking. Write these goals down in a diary or on your phone and track your progress. Celebrate your wins, no matter how small, and adjust your targets as you grow stronger and more confident.

Make daily tasks active: Convert mundane tasks into opportunities for movement
Turning everyday moments into movement can be easy. For examples, the next time you are chatting on the phone, why not walk around your room or garden? It is a great way to keep the body active. When you are settled in for some television time, those ad breaks are the perfect time to stand up, stretch out, or do a few gentle exercises. These minor changes will not disrupt your routine, but can make a significant difference in keeping your body moving and your heart pumping.

Listen to your body
Tuning into the way you feel is important. If you are feeling energetic, it might be a good day to challenge yourself with a longer walk or an additional exercise routine. On days when tiredness or discomfort creep in, it is okay to ease up and choose gentler activities (or even rest).

>> ACTION POINTS - PRIORITY 2 <<

Weekly goals

Start by jotting down what you would like to achieve: it could be walking 5,000 steps a day, having two yoga sessions, or climbing the stairs for 5 minutes a day. Make these goals SMART and specific to your lifestyle. Place this list somewhere visible as a daily reminder and each week, review how you have done, and adjust accordingly based on your comfort and progress.

Desk exercises

Staying active at your desk can be simple and effective - during breaks, try seated leg lifts or ankle circles to keep blood flowing. Gently stretch your neck from side to side or roll your shoulders backwards to ease tension. Every hour, stand and reach up, elongating your spine.

Utilise breaks effectively: If you are working, use breaks as an opportunity to move

To maximise your breaks, set a regular timer – perhaps every hour – as a reminder to move. When it sounds, stand up, stretch out your limbs, or even take a short walk outside. You need little; just a few minutes of movement can do wonders.

>> ADDRESSING CHALLENGES <<

While integrating movement can be straightforward, it can feel challenging at times, and here are some common obstacles you might come up against, and how to address them:

Lack of time: The perception of not having enough time
Feeling that you lack time to exercise is often about perspective. So rather than viewing activity as an extra chore, embed it within your daily tasks. You could stand while taking a call, use the farthest toilet at work, or do calf raises while cooking. Make the most of the movements and activities that you already do.

Physical limitations: You might have health issues or physical limitations that restrict movement
Foremost, seek advice from your doctor or personal trainer to understand what is safe for you. They can recommend tailored activities that align with your capabilities. It might be gentle seated exercises, resistance bands, or guided stretches. The goal is to keep moving within your comfort zone and ability, embracing the activities that suit you and maintaining a regular rhythm.

Lack of motivation: Building new habits requires motivation
Feeling unmotivated can be a hurdle, but it is one you can overcome. Start by pinpointing what activities you enjoy - be it dancing, walking, or even gardening. Once identified, set clear, achievable goals related

to this activity and keep a simple log to track your progress. Watching your own advancements can be incredibly motivating, so embrace the fun side of movement; it is about feeling good, both mentally and physically

Walking

Walking regularly and gradually increasing your daily step count can benefit your physical and mental health. It is very underrated and often overlooked as an exercise.

Walking is great for all ages and fitness levels as it is low impact, requires no special equipment and can be done pretty much anywhere. The gentle, rhythmic act of walking can help with weight loss, can improve cardiovascular health, and can also have a positive impact on blood sugar levels by improving the efficiency of your muscles' ability to utilise glucose.

While walking might not seem like an intense calorie-burning exercise, it is the consistency and duration that matter. Taking a 30-minute walk after meals can burn calories and help with weight management - which is important for preventing and reversing type 2 diabetes. Walking can improve circulation, reduces bad cholesterol levels, and can keep blood pressure in check. Over time, it strengthens the entire cardiovascular system.

Make walking a regular part of your daily routine - even if it is just for a few minutes a day.

>> ACTION POINTS - PRIORITY 1 <<

Start small: If you are new to regular walking, aim for a comfortable 10-minute stroll

Taking those first steps towards a walking routine need not be daunting. Pop on a pair of trainers or suitable shoes and venture out for a relaxed 10-minute walk around your neighbourhood. After a few days, challenge yourself to add an extra 30 seconds or a minute each time. No pressure, just go with what feels right.

Stay hydrated: Carry a bottle of water with you

Walking increases fluid loss from your body so, before you head out, fill a water bottle, and take it with you. As you walk, take regular sips, especially on warmer days or longer routes. Do not wait until you are thirsty to drink; instead, make it a habit to sip little and often.

Listen to your body: Stay in tune with your body's signals

During your walks, maintain a gentle awareness of how you feel. If something does not seem right – be it a twinge in your knee or a slight breathlessness – do not push through; instead, slow down or take a brief rest.

Monitor blood sugar: Walking can influence blood sugar levels

The act of walking can affect blood sugar levels. Before going out, take a quick moment to check your blood sugar using a home monitor. This ensures you are starting from a safe baseline. When you return from your walk, test again to observe any changes. This habit helps you understand your body's reactions to walking, enabling you to tweak the length or pace of your walks.

>> ACTION POINTS - PRIORITY 2 <<

Mix it up: Walking need not be monotonous

Each week, pick a day to venture somewhere new. This simple change not only refreshes your mind, but can also engage different muscles. During your walk, try incorporating moments of brisk walking with periods of relaxed pace. These minor variations can uplift your mood, enhance cardiovascular benefits, and keep every walk feeling like a new adventure.

Post-meal walks: Incorporate a gentle 10-15 minute walk after your meals

Embracing a short stroll after meals is a great way to support your body. By dedicating 10-15 minutes post-meal to wander around your local area or garden, you will assist your body to process glucose more efficiently. Remember, it is not about pace, but consistency.

Strength Training

Strength training (also known as resistance training) can be a useful tool in your blood sugar control toolbox. At its basic level, it is simply exercise that uses weight or resistance to make your muscles work harder than they would normally do.

You don't have to go to the gym or buy expensive equipment to build muscle. Basic exercises using your body weight or common household items can be just as effective and motivate you to exercise regularly.

There are some very specific benefits to strength training in preventing or reversing type 2 diabetes. Strength training increases the energy needs of your muscles, causing them to use more glucose from your blood, lowering your blood sugar levels. In addition, training regularly can make muscle cells better at absorbing glucose and insulin sensitivity can improve.

The benefits of strength training go far beyond blood sugar control though, as it can help in weight management (by building muscle) which can improve your metabolism. It can also help you burn visceral fat (the deep abdominal fat around the organs associated with type 2 diabetes and cardiovascular problems), stimulate the growth of bone tissue (which reduces the risk of osteoporosis and bone fractures, particularly as we age), it can have a positive impact on your mental health (reducing feelings of depression or anxiety), and it can boost your self-esteem.

Strength training can fit it easily into your day-to-day life. As I have mentioned, it does not require heavy weights or gym memberships. Simple bodyweight exercises, like squats or push-ups, or using household items as weights can be just as effective. The key is consistency and progression.

>> ACTION POINTS - PRIORITY 1 <<

Start slowly: If you are new to strength training, seek professional guidance
Starting your strength training journey? Take it slow, hire a trainer, and start with lighter weights to get the hang of the exercises. Proper form is pivotal, not just for the workout's efficacy, but to reduce the risk of injuries.

Consistency: Aim for regularity and consistency in your training sessions
The key to consistency in strength training is developing a habit of steady rhythm, rather than sporadic intensity. Aim to set aside dedicated days and times for your sessions, allowing it to become a natural part of your routine.

Monitor blood sugar: If you have type 2 diabetes, it is advisable to check blood sugar levels before and after exercise (especially in the early stages)

When embarking on strength training, understanding how exercise impacts your blood sugar is key. By checking your blood sugar levels before a workout, you ensure you are starting from a safe baseline. Post-exercise checks help gauge how your body has responded to that specific activity. This monitoring helps you achieve a balance between strength gains and stable blood sugar levels during workouts.

Stay hydrated: Ensure you drink adequate water before, during and after your session

Proper hydration is essential. To integrate this into your routine, make it a habit to drink a glass of water about 30 minutes before starting and keep a water bottle within reach during your session, taking small sips regularly. It acts as a reminder to pause, breathe, and hydrate. Once you have wrapped up, drink another glass to aid in recovery.

Warm-up and cool down: Begin each session with a 5-10 minute warm-up phase, and end with a cool-down phase

Begin by doing 5-10 minutes of light aerobic exercises like brisk walking or cycling to get your heart rate up. This prepares your muscles and joints for the activity ahead. Once your session is complete, do not rush off; dedicate another 5-10 minutes and gently stretch each muscle group you have worked on. The cool-down phase helps relax your muscles, reduce stiffness, and prepare your body for the next session, ensuring safe and effective training.

Rest and recovery: Allow your muscles to recover by giving at least one day of rest between strength training sessions

In the world of strength training, rest is where the magic happens. When you lift weights, you are creating tiny tears in your muscles. These tears rebuild stronger during rest days, leading to muscle growth. To put this action point into practice, simply schedule your strength training sessions with at least a day's gap in between. For instance, if you train on a Monday, your next session could be on Wednesday. During your off days, engage in light activities or stretching if you fancy, but avoid intense muscle-specific workouts. Remember, it is during the rest that your muscles grow and repair.

>> ACTION POINT - PRIORITY 2 <<

Diversify: Incorporate a mix of bodyweight exercises, free weights and resistance bands

Diversifying your strength training keeps it interesting and effectively targets different muscle groups. Squats or push-ups, utilise your natural weight, making them accessible anytime. Free weights, such as dumbbells, offer versatility in movement and intensity. Resistance bands, being portable and adaptable, provide tension that challenges muscles in unique ways. By combining these elements, you get a well-rounded workout that prevents boredom and boosts strength.

Cardiovascular Exercise

Cardiovascular exercise (cardio) raises your heart and your breathing rate and engages the large muscle groups without the need for weights. Cardio has several benefits, such as strengthening the heart, improving blood circulation, enhancing respiratory efficiency, and releasing endorphins for pain relief and mood improvement. Cardio promotes better sleep patterns and helps with weight management when paired with a balanced diet.

When it comes to managing blood sugar, cardio exercises increase muscle sensitivity to insulin and use glucose for muscle repair, resulting in lower blood sugar levels.

Walking (as covered in the previous section) is a good example of a low-impact type of cardio workout and is great for beginners. Cycling (whether stationary or outdoor) offers an excellent cardio workout with lesser impact on the knees and joints. Swimming is a great way to workout your whole body, improve heart health, and tone muscles without hurting your joints. Dancing is a fun way to elevate the heart rate (whether it is ballroom, salsa, or a simple dance fitness class, dancing can be both enjoyable and effective).

>> ACTION POINTS - PRIORITY 1 <<

Start slow: If you are new to cardio exercise, begin with shorter, less intense sessions

It is important to begin with sessions that are manageable for your current fitness level. Perhaps start with a ten-minute brisk walk, then each week, add another few minutes. As your endurance builds, you can then introduce more challenging activities or intensify your current ones. By following this method, you can ensure your safety, avoid injuries, and establish a sustainable exercise routine at a comfortable pace.

Stay hydrated: Regularly drink water before, during and after your workout

For better performance and recovery during cardio workouts, drink a glass of water 30 minutes before you start. During your session, especially if it is prolonged or in warm conditions, sip water at intervals to replace the fluids you are losing through sweat. Post-workout, drink another glass to ensure you are re-hydrating. Remember, thirst is not always an immediate indicator, so make drinking water a consistent part of your exercise routine.

Wear the right footwear: Support your feet and reduce the risk of injury

Proper footwear will meet the specific demands of your activity by providing support, cushioning, and stability. It is worthwhile visiting a specialised sports shop where staff can guide you based on your foot type and gait. Investing in quality shoes not only enhances comfort but also minimises the strain on your joints, reducing the risk of potential injuries. Remember, comfort and safety are paramount.

Listen to your body: Understand the difference between 'good pain' (like muscle soreness) and 'bad pain' (like joint pain or chest discomfort)
It is important to be in tune with your body's signals. Feeling sore muscles after a good workout can be a normal part of building strength, but sharp pains, joint discomfort, or any unusual chest sensations should not be overlooked. These might indicate something more serious, so if you experience what feels like 'bad pain', it is essential to halt your activity and consult your doctor. It is always better to be safe than sorry, rather than push through and potentially worsen an issue.

>> ACTION POINTS - PRIORITY 2 <<

Create a routine: Set a schedule that fits into your daily life and stick to it
Start by setting specific days and times in your week for exercise to make it easier to prioritise your cardiovascular workouts. Choose moments when you feel most energetic and motivated, whether that is a morning jog or an evening dance class. Once set, treat these time slots as non-negotiable - much like an important appointment. Consistency not only builds discipline but also ensures you reap the long-term

benefits of your efforts.

Mix it up: Engage in a variety of cardio workouts to keep things interesting

Instead of doing the same activity every day, like jogging, try switching it up by cycling, swimming, or joining a dance class. This approach improves endurance, challenges various muscles, and prevents boredom. Different workouts offer different advantages - swimming is easy on the joints, while dancing improves coordination.

Enjoy nature: Whenever possible, choose outdoor sessions

Embracing nature while doing cardio has dual benefits - it is good for your mental health and your physical health.

Household Tasks: Movement in Disguise

Daily around-the-home chores are often seen as mundane tasks that we need to check off our to-do lists as soon as possible, but these can be helpful in increasing activity levels.

Routine household jobs, from sweeping floors to tending to the garden, encapsulate movement in its most natural form. When observed through the lens of health and in the context of blood sugar control, these daily activities can transform into powerful tools.

Vacuuming and sweeping engage your core and arm muscles, providing a mini workout. Activities like digging, planting and even mowing the lawn are excellent ways to incorporate movement. Washing the car or general around the house cleaning also gives your limbs a good stretch and workout.

Yes, your household chores can play a key role in keeping you physically active - and common jobs around the home such as vacuuming, mopping or even rearranging furniture can burn significant calories. While these figures might not be quite the same as a strenuous gym session, they are still valuable and still count.

Many chores also engage various muscle groups. For example: lifting laundry baskets can engage the arm and back muscles, while squatting to pick up items can work the leg muscles. Over time, these movements contribute to muscle tone and strength. Doing tasks that involve stretching or reaching, like dusting high shelves or washing windows, naturally increases flexibility.

Being active within your own personal limitations plays a key role in blood sugar control, and household chores offer a low-impact, accessible way to keep moving (which is especially beneficial for those who might find exercise regimes challenging). As we have established, physical activity helps in using up glucose for energy, which can contribute to better blood sugar levels. Regular activity (even if it is through daily chores) can assist in weight management.

And finally, completing household tasks can give you a sense of accomplishment. When coupled with the physical activity aspect, they can release our natural mood lifters, endorphins, and potentially help to reduce the stress that often comes with managing a chronic condition.

>> ACTION POINTS - PRIORITY 1 <<

Mindfulness in movement: Being present in the moment and consciously engaging with the task can make it more enjoyable and efficient
The next time you are vacuuming or tidying, take a moment to focus on

your movements. Feel the stretch in your arms as you reach, or the stability in your legs as you bend. Pay attention to your posture — are your shoulders relaxed, is your back straight? By being present, not only will you make the task more enjoyable, but you also ensure that you are moving in ways that benefit your body, supporting both your physical health and your diabetes management journey.

Regular breaks: If you have a lot to tackle, ensure you take short breaks to stretch or hydrate

While tackling your household chores, set a gentle reminder, perhaps on your phone or kitchen timer, for every 30 minutes. When it rings, pause your activity, take a moment to stretch out any tense muscles and perhaps enjoy a small glass of water. This little habit not only offers your body a brief respite, but it also keeps you hydrated and ensures you are integrating movement into your day.

>> ACTION POINT - PRIORITY 2 <<

Rotate tasks: To engage different muscle groups, rotate between tasks

When planning your household chores, consider grouping them in pairs that use different parts of your body. Start with tasks like dusting or wiping surfaces, then switch to activities like mopping or vacuuming. This rotation method not only breaks the monotony but also ensures you are giving various muscles a workout.

Step 2 Summary

Phew! The physicality of step 2 can be quite challenging, particularly if you are not used to much regular movement or exercise. I trust you have noted down some action points that you plan to start working on straight away. Don't forget, any movement is better than no movement at all - so if you are very sedentary and from today take a 10-minute walk around the block, then that is a great way to start. If you are already going to your local gym but only once or twice a month at the moment but now have decided to go once a week, then kudos to you.

Movement can have a positive reinforcing loop effect. The more you do regularly (even if it is a 10-minute stroll) then the more you will feel and see benefits. The more you feel and see benefits, then the more you will probably do. Embrace movement. It is an important factor in preventing and reversing type 2 diabetes.

Remember, you can schedule a free 15-minute Zoom or phone session with me at **www.diabetessolutions.co.uk/support-sessions** for additional help or a confidential chat about your progress.

To prevent or reverse type 2 diabetes, diet and exercise are key areas that often need to be changed and improved. In step 3, we are going to build on what you have learnt so far, and look at the 'less tangible' but equally important areas of your wellbeing; including your mental health, sleep quality, stress management, and more. Every one of the areas covered in step 3 has as much an intrinsic value to your health as everything covered so far in steps 1 and 2.

So, pen at the ready! There are lots more juicy action points to be worked on in the following step - so let's dive in!

Step 3: Holistic Wellbeing

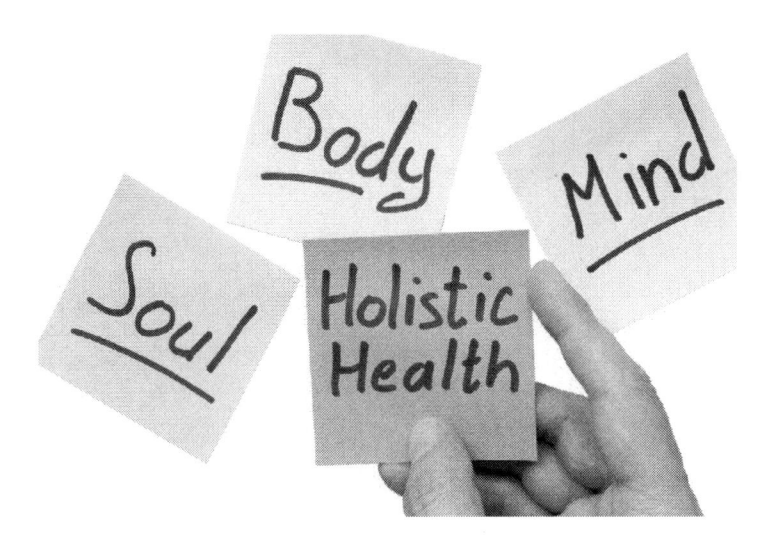

Introduction

Welcome to Step 3 - Holistic Wellbeing

In step 1, we looked at diet and nutrition. In step 2, we reviewed the importance of physical movement in relation to blood sugar control.

As we have now covered diet, nutrition, and exercise, you might assume that is all that needs to be known about preventing or reversing type 2 diabetes. Indeed, you might expect me to begin concluding the book at this point.

But you would be incorrect. Please allow me to explain why...

Yes, preventing and reversing type 2 diabetes has a lot to do with diet - of course it does: "You are what you eat", as the saying goes. Your diet will, for the most part, determine whether you develop type 2 diabetes (in the short, medium or long term) or if you already have it, whether you might reverse it. Then comes movement and exercise and yes, activity is important - those with a sedentary lifestyle not only increase their risk of developing type 2 diabetes, but a range of other health problems too.

So why am I not concluding my book after covering these key factors? Because preventing or reversing the type 2 diabetes goes beyond simply what you eat and how much you move. It also involves your mind, your thought processes, your psychology, your stress management, your sleep quality and more. In fact, I would argue that to be successful in prevention or reversal, what goes on between your ears is as equally (if not more) important than the types of calories you eat or the number of steps you do each day.

Time to grab your pen and your 'Action Points' worksheet from your bonus pack. There is still much to uncover.

The Mind-Body Connection

Your body is remarkable, and so too is your mind. But often they are seen as two separate entities when, in fact, they are deeply interwoven with each other. The relationship between your mental and physical health is intrinsically connected, and understanding this connection is important.

Being 'healthy' involves more than just diet and exercise - we need to look at elements of your mental wellbeing too. This section is not a detailed exploration of psychology and psychiatry, but it will provide you with a basic understanding of the topic.

Let us first look at the body > mind connection.

You may wonder how your physical health can have an influence on your mental state. Just think about a day when you've had plenty of sleep, a nourishing meal, and a pleasant walk - typically, your mood is better, your patience lasts longer, and you see life in a more positive light. Now flip that coin and think of a day filled with physical discomfort, perhaps because of an ailment or fatigue and a poor night's sleep. On such days, irritability, a lack of focus, or feelings of sadness might overshadow your experiences.

When it comes to your heart, good cardiovascular health helps the efficient delivery of essential nutrients to the brain. If your cardiovascular health is compromised, it can decrease oxygen flow to the brain and affect your cognitive abilities and mood.

Let us not overlook the importance of good gut health either, as this plays a significant role in your mental wellbeing. A well-functioning digestive system and healthy gut bacteria ensures you absorb nutrients efficiently, which plays a vital role in your brain function. Did you know, for example, that the absorption of essential fatty acids, amino acids and certain minerals directly impacts neurotransmitter functions in the brain - those that are responsible for mood regulation?

The physical state of your body can dictate your mood through biochemical means, too. For example, physical activity prompts the release of endorphins, often termed "feel-good" hormones, which can ease feelings of sadness or depression.

Now, let us examine the mind > body link.

We all love a good night's sleep, don't we? Well, quality sleep is one of the cornerstones of both good physical and mental health, as it ensures bodily repair, immune function optimisation, and toxin removal. When you are well-rested, your mental clarity improves, and you are better equipped to handle stress. On the other hand, disrupted or inadequate sleep can lead to mood swings, irritability, a heightened sense of stress and often bad food choices as you get the 'munchies' and seek those sugary carbohydrate goodies to snack on.

Your psychological state often dictates the daily choices you make, which impacts your physical health. When you feel motivated and positive, you are more inclined to exercise, eat healthily, and stay away from harmful habits. On the flip side, if you are feeling depressed or have a low mood, you might turn to overeating, inactivity, or relying on substances, which can have consequences for your health.

Stress is often considered a mental or emotional response to a situation, and it has tangible physical outcomes. When you are anxious, upset, or overwhelmed, your body releases the stress hormones epinephrine (adrenaline), cortisol, and norepinephrin. While these hormones serve a purpose in immediate "fight or flight" situations, chronic exposure can lead to elevated blood pressure, digestive issues, and blood sugar rises.

There is increasing evidence that shows how your emotional state can influence your immunity, too. Consistent feelings of hopelessness or depression can weaken your immune system, making you more susceptible to getting sick. Conversely, positivity and emotional resilience can strengthen your immune response.

Mindfulness, meditation and other mental wellness practices, while primarily focusing on the mind, also have physical advantages. By engaging in these practices, you can experience lower blood pressure, better digestion, and improved blood sugar control. They work by mitigating the body's stress response, resulting in tangible physical health benefits. We will look at these in more detail shortly.

>> ACTION POINTS - PRIORITY 1 <<

Regular check-ins: Routinely assessing your mental and physical wellbeing is essential

Regularly pause and tune in to how you are feeling, both mentally and physically. Maybe keep a simple journal, noting down how you are feeling and any changes in your body. If something feels not quite right, it is okay to seek help.

Rest and rejuvenate: Ensure adequate sleep

To ensure a good night's rest, set a regular bedtime and stick to it (even on weekends). Create a calming bedtime routine: perhaps a warm bath, a cup of herbal tea, or some light reading. Ensure your sleeping environment is cool, dark, and quiet. If you find your mind racing, try gentle breathing exercises to help you relax.

Self-reflection: Regularly assess your mental state and acknowledge feelings, understanding they have physical implications

Checking in with your mental wellbeing is just as vital as monitoring your physical health. Every day, find a calm moment to ask yourself, "How am I feeling today?" Identify and label these emotions without being harsh on yourself and realise that your feelings can impact your physical health, possibly affecting your blood sugar levels or your food choices. By acknowledging your emotions, you are in a stronger position to take proactive steps for both mental and physical wellness.

Embrace mindfulness: Allocate at least 10 minutes daily for mindfulness or meditation

Adding mindfulness (which we will cover shortly) to your daily routine is good for your mental and physical health. Start by setting aside a dedicated 10 minutes each day, perhaps in the morning or before bed. Find a quiet space, sit comfortably, and focus on your breathing and let go of the day's stresses, bringing your attention to the present moment.

Prioritise physical activity: Regular exercise can improve both your mental and physical health

Incorporating exercise into your routine need not be daunting. Begin with small steps, perhaps a 10-minute brisk walk daily and over time, gradually increase the duration or add variety like cycling or swimming. Regular activity not only helps regulate blood sugar but also releases endorphins, your 'feel-good' hormones. Remember, it is consistency over intensity; find an activity you enjoy and stick with it.

Evaluate your diet: Recognise the influence of dietary choices on both blood sugar levels and mental wellbeing

Keep a simple food diary for a week, noting down your meals and any mood or energy shifts afterwards. Soon, patterns may emerge linking certain foods with energy spikes or mood changes and then, armed with this insight, you can tweak your diet, favouring foods that stabilise blood sugar and uplift your mood.

>> ACTION POINTS - PRIORITY 2 <<

Celebrate small wins: Regularly acknowledge and celebrate your progress, however small, to maintain motivation and mental wellbeing

Recognising your achievements boosts your spirits and keeps you on track - so start by setting tangible, achievable goals. Each time you reach one, take a moment to appreciate your effort. Perhaps it is a gratitude journal entry, a special (non-food!) treat or simply sharing with a friend. Celebrating small victories not only uplifts your mood, but also reinforces your commitment to your goals.

Seek support: Whether it is from loved ones, support groups, or professionals - it is good to have a support system in place

Start by opening up to close friends or family about your goals and concerns. If you prefer, there are many support groups, both online and in the community, catering to various health needs. For personalised advice, considering reaching out to a suitable professional. Everyone's journey is unique, but having a supportive shoulder or a listening ear can make all the difference in nurturing your mind-body relationship.

Empowering the Mind for Physical Healing

As we saw in the previous section, your mind holds significant sway over your physical health. While this has been understood this for many years, scientific research now offers concrete insights into just how the mind influences bodily functions.

One of the most studied phenomena showcasing the mind's power is the placebo effect. Patients can show improvements in their conditions simply by believing in the treatment, even if they were given a harmless sugar pill. The mind's expectation of healing can indeed cause actual physical healing.

One of the first steps in harnessing mental strength is clarity and setting clear intentions like "I will maintain stable blood sugar levels" or "I will lead an active lifestyle". By so doing, you lay the foundation to focus your mental energies on guiding your actions.

Visualisation is a powerful tool for mentally rehearsing the achievement of a desired outcome, such as picturing yourself engaging in a morning walk or imagining a day filled with making good food and drink choices. By visualising positive scenarios repeatedly, you can mentally prepare for them, making it easier to put them into action.

Positive affirmations (concise and positive statements declared as if they are already true) can help shape your subconscious thinking. Statements like "I am in control of my health" or "every day, I make choices that benefit my wellbeing" can offer a boost of motivation and foster a proactive approach to the day ahead.

While the power of the mind is immense, it can pose challenges. Sometimes, mental barriers from beliefs or past experiences can block your progress. At some point, we've all believed things like "I can't control my cravings" or "exercise is too challenging." Acknowledging and accepting these beliefs is the first step in getting rid of them.

Once we identify such beliefs, the next step is reframing. Instead of saying "I cannot control my cravings", you might say "every day, I am learning better ways to manage my diet".

>> ACTION POINTS - PRIORITY 1 <<

Journaling: Regularly jot down your thoughts, feelings, and intentions

Begin with a simple notebook and each day, take a few moments to write down your feelings, experiences, and intentions. This does not need to be lengthy; sometimes a sentence or two can capture your mindset and, over time, you will see patterns and become attuned to your emotional triggers and strengths. This self-awareness guides you in reshaping any unhelpful beliefs and bolsters those that empower you.

Daily visualisation: Dedicate a few minutes every day to visualise your health goals and the steps you need to take to achieve them

Begin by finding a quiet spot, free from distractions, and then close your eyes and vividly imagine your health goals. See yourself achieving them, feeling vibrant and full of energy. Focus not just on the end result, but also on the positive actions you are taking each day towards this vision. Feel the emotions associated with success. By regularly immersing yourself in this visual journey, you are making your health goals feel more achievable.

Use affirmations: Start your day with positive affirmations

Each morning, after waking up, find a calm moment to state a positive affirmation aloud, such as "every day, I am making choices that benefit my health." Speak with conviction and believe in the words you are saying. This not only sets a positive tone for the day, but also reinforces your commitment. These daily declarations can help you develop a resilient and optimistic mindset for tackling challenges.

Celebrate milestones: Recognise and celebrate your progress, no matter how minor

Start by setting tangible, achievable goals related to your health and, whenever you hit one, take a moment to acknowledge your effort. It could be as simple as treating yourself to a favourite book, taking a day off for relaxation, or enjoying a nice warm bath. Remember, every step forward, no matter its size, is an achievement. By celebrating the small victories, you are not only boosting your resolve but also reinforcing the positive habits that led you there.

>> ACTION POINTS - PRIORITY 2 <<

Seek support: Consider joining support groups
Research local or online support groups centred around health and wellness (or any specific challenges you are facing). These groups offer a safe space to share experiences and learn from others. If you feel you might benefit from additional help, then consider reaching out to a qualified therapist who can provide tailored guidance.

Meditation: A few minutes of daily meditation can help in reducing stress and reinforcing positive intentions
To integrate meditation into your routine, find a quiet spot in your home. Sit comfortably, close your eyes, and focus on your breathing. Even just 5 minutes daily can make a difference. As thoughts arise, gently bring your attention back to your breath. Over time, you will notice enhanced calmness and clarity, which can positively influence your health journey. If unsure where to start, there are many free guided sessions online tailored for beginners.

Mindful Eating

Did you know that the 'how' of eating can be just as consequential as the 'what'?

An unusual statement I know, but while we know that choosing healthy foods is important for our diet and blood sugar control, how we eat our meals is also vital.

This is known as 'mindful eating'.

Mindful eating is a practice that encourages us to form a stronger connection with our food - for us to be present in the moment of eating, savouring the food and listening to our bodies.

The essence of mindful eating lies in consciously focusing on the experience of eating and drinking. It entails observing the colours, textures and aromas of your food, as well as recognising how it makes you feel and the signals your body sends about taste, satisfaction and fullness.

Mindful eating can also offer you insights into how certain foods impact your blood sugar levels, your energy and your overall wellbeing. Instead of gulping down a meal in the quickest possible time and with the fewest chews as possible (and then realising too late that you have overeaten, chosen foods that cause a sugar spike or now have indigestion) mindful eating encourages a more measured, conscious approach.

There are many benefits to practising mindful eating:
- Improved blood sugar control (as by paying attention to how foods affect your energy and satiety, you can make better decisions about portion sizes and food choices),
- Enhanced satisfaction from the food you eat (when you savour each bite, you get more pleasure from lesser amounts of food),
- Reducing stress related to eating (instead of worrying about what you 'should' or 'should not' eat, you develop a healthier relationship with food and eating becomes an act of self-care),
- Better digestion and overall health (as eating slowly and deliberately can aid digestion, allowing you to absorb the maximum nutrients from your food).

It is easy to integrate mindful eating into your daily routine by following these four steps:
1. **Silence:** Before you begin your meal, take a few moments, as this can help in setting a calm atmosphere, and make you more in tune with your food.
2. **Engagement:** Observe the colours on your plate, smell the aromas, relish the textures, and allow yourself to truly experience your food.
3. **Chewing:** Not only does this aid digestion, but it also gives you the time to savour each bite.

4. **Observing:** Begin recognising hunger and fullness cues and ask yourself if you are eating because you are genuinely hungry or is it out of habit, boredom or emotion?

Mindful eating may seem simple, but it' is challenging to practise regularly in our busy lives. Distractions like our modern day electronic devices, the television and even work can detract from your eating experience - and it may take you a little time to cultivate this habit. Remember that every meal is a new opportunity to practise mindfulness and if you find your mind wandering during meals, gently bring your focus back to the food. If external distractions are an issue, create an environment conducive to mindful eating: turn off electronics and the TV, play calming music, or simply enjoy the sounds of nature if you are dining outdoors.

>> ACTION POINTS - PRIORITY 1 <<

Practice regularly: Aim for at least one mindful meal a day
Start small, perhaps with breakfast or a snack. Choose a meal where you can spare a few quiet moments. Dedicate this time solely to eating, noticing the flavours, textures and how you feel. Over the coming days and weeks, this small window of mindfulness will become a habit and you will find that, even on busy days, it will be easier to find moments to eat mindfully. Remember, it is not about perfection, but consistent practice.

Set the stage: For your next meal, create an environment free of distractions

Choose a quiet place for your meal and clear away any clutter from where you are about to eat. Switch off the TV, your mobile phone, or any other distractions and as you sit down, take a moment to appreciate the aroma and appearance of your food. Let yourself be fully present, savouring each bite, noticing the textures and flavours.

Be kind to yourself: If you find yourself slipping back into old habits, do not berate yourself

Embracing mindfulness is part of the journey, not a destination - so if you notice old habits creeping in, take a gentle pause. Rather than criticising or berating yourself, acknowledge the moment and use it as a reminder to refocus. Think of each meal as a chance to improve your mindfulness.

>> ACTION POINT - PRIORITY 2 <<

Journal the experience: After eating mindfully, jot down your feelings, observations and your body's reactions

Taking a moment after your meal to reflect can be enlightening. Keep a dedicated journal nearby and after you have finished eating, jot down a few lines about how the food made you feel, any specific tastes you noticed and how your body reacted. Did you feel satisfied, perhaps energised? By documenting your food habits, you can make better choices and develop a healthier relationship with food.

The Importance Of Sleep

Sleep is considered by many to be a passive activity. We go to bed, we fall asleep, and we wake up in the morning - completely unaware of the complex processes that have been going on overnight. Some people do not realise that sleep is crucial for health, so they intentionally get very little or even less than the minimum amount needed to maintain good health.

Sleep deprivation can have a serious impact on physical and mental health and on blood sugar levels, too. It is an important subject in relation to type 2 diabetes and blood sugar control, so let's dig a little deeper and find out why quality and quantity of sleep is so important.

Lack of sleep is a type of stress and, when stressed, the body releases cortisol (the stress hormone). Persistently elevated cortisol levels can lead to reduced insulin sensitivity - which can make blood sugar control challenging.

Extended periods of poor sleep (either in terms of quality or quantity, or both) can lead to an increase in free fatty acids in the bloodstream, and these fatty acids can interfere with glucose metabolism, further contributing to higher blood sugar levels. Chronic sleep deprivation can also start an inflammatory response in the body, and this state of low-level inflammation can make the body less responsive to insulin too.

The Sleep Cycle
Each cycle lasts 90-110 minutes

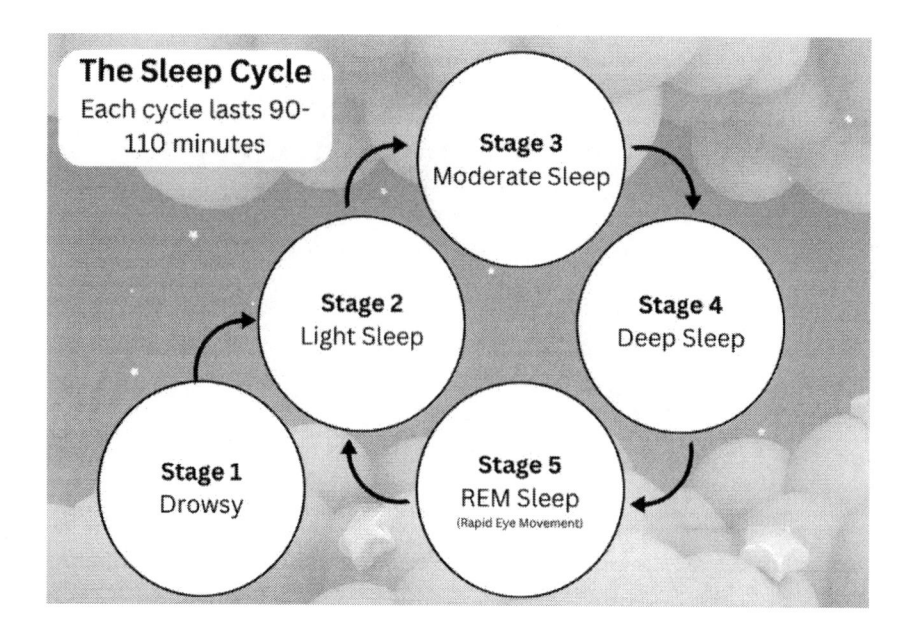

- Stage 1 Drowsy
- Stage 2 Light Sleep
- Stage 3 Moderate Sleep
- Stage 4 Deep Sleep
- Stage 5 REM Sleep (Rapid Eye Movement)

During deep sleep, growth hormone is released, and it plays several roles - one of which is how the body processes glucose. Without adequate deep sleep, the expected surge of growth hormone is curtailed, potentially leading to less effective glucose processing and subsequent elevated blood sugar levels.

A good night's sleep helps to regulate ghrelin (known as the 'hunger hormone', and that signals to our brain that it is time to eat) and leptin (the hormone that sends messages to the brain to signal that we are full). Lack of sleep increases ghrelin levels and decreases leptin levels - and this imbalance can lead to increased hunger and appetite, often for sugary or high-carbohydrate foods, which then increases blood sugar levels and, in the long term, can contribute to weight gain.

Insulin assists cells in absorbing sugar, while glucagon signals the liver to release stored sugar. These hormones are regulated during the night. Lack of sleep can throw off this balance and cause higher blood sugar levels in the morning.

Many of us will have the odd bad night's sleep due to stress, what we ate or drank the evening before, and many other reasons. It is important to understand that it is not just one bad night's sleep that we need to be concerned about. It is chronic sleep disruptions or consistently shortened sleep cycles that are of concern and that can create a cumulative effect, progressively impairing the body's ability to regulate blood sugar effectively.

The Sleep > Stress > Sugar Link

Stress is, at its core, the body's response to any change or challenge, requiring an adjustment or reaction. It is a primal reaction that has evolved as a means of survival and while acute stress is a natural part of life, chronic or prolonged stress can become detrimental to your health, including your metabolic health.

The connection between stress, sleep and sugar metabolism is complex, and can be visualised as a triangle, where each point influences the next.

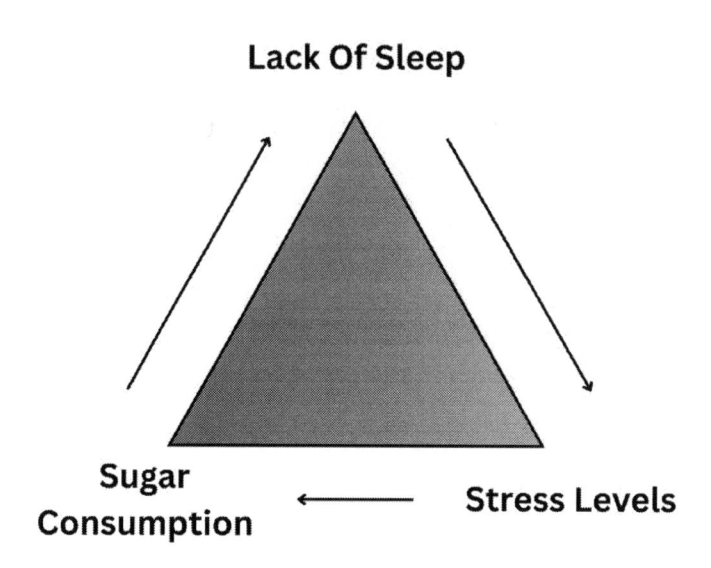

Lack Of Sleep

Sugar Consumption ⟵ **Stress Levels**

A lack of sleep is a stressor. When you do not get enough sleep, your body's stress hormone - cortisol – rises. Having consistently high cortisol levels can lead to health issues, such as problems with blood sugar regulation.

Prolonged stress, whether from lack of sleep or other sources, can lead to increased blood sugar levels. The body, under stress, releases extra energy as glucose to prepare for the 'fight or flight' response. However, when this energy is not used, it results in raised blood sugar levels. High blood sugar levels can cause nighttime urination and nerve pain, disrupting sleep patterns.

It is easy to see how this negative loop can emerge: lack of sleep increases stress, stress raises blood sugar levels and then high blood sugar can further disturb sleep. Breaking this cycle becomes crucial for those with or at risk of type 2 diabetes.

Quality sleep provides the body and mind with an opportunity to recover from your stresses of the day. When you sleep, your body repairs cells, consolidates memories, and processes emotions, which can lower stress levels.

Chronic sleep deprivation has been linked to mood disturbances, including irritability, anxiety, and depression. Ensuring a good night's sleep can help improve your emotional health, enabling you to better handle stressful situations. Adequate sleep assists in regulating hormones connected to hunger, satisfaction, and stress, resulting in a more balanced metabolic state.

Techniques like mindfulness and meditation can help you remain present, can help to reduce stress, and can cultivate a more positive connection between your mind and your body. Reinforcing positive thoughts can improve your blood sugar control. Speaking with a CBT professional can help you understand the connection between your thoughts, feelings, and behaviours, enabling you to make better health decisions.

So now you can see the importance that sleep has, to your physical, mental, and emotional health, and also your blood sugar levels. By working towards consistent, high-quality sleep, you can steady the delicate balance of hormones that influence your appetite, stress levels, and blood sugar.

>> ACTION POINTS - PRIORITY 1 <<

Establish a routine: Set a regular sleep schedule, where you go to bed and wake up at the same time every day
Start by choosing a bedtime and wake-up time that suits your lifestyle and daily commitments. Stick to these times diligently, even on weekends. Over a few days, you will probably notice your body naturally feeling sleepy or waking up around those times.

Create a restful environment: Your bedroom should be a sanctuary for sleep
To craft a sleep-conducive bedroom, focus on three key elements: darkness, silence, and temperature. Begin by hanging blackout curtains to block any external light. If street noise or household sounds disturb your sleep, consider investing in a white noise machine or earplugs to create a serene soundscape. Lastly, aim to keep the room cool – most find a temperature of around 18°C optimal.

Be mindful of diet: What you eat can influence sleep
Diet plays a pivotal role in sleep quality and quantity, so consider

having a lighter evening meal and finishing it a couple of hours before you go to bed. If you are sipping on a cup of tea or coffee, switch to decaffeinated versions by mid-afternoon at the latest. And while a glass of wine or a couple of beers might feel relaxing, alcohol can hinder deep sleep phases. If you are regularly getting up in the night to go to the toilet, perhaps stop consuming fluids an hour or two before retiring to bed.

Avoid harmful coping mechanisms: Refrain from using substances like excessive alcohol to cope

When faced with stress, it is essential to choose healthy coping strategies. If you are tempted to use alcohol or other substances, try to redirect that urge towards more positive outlets and engage in activities you love, be it reading, listening to music, or taking a walk. Stay connected with loved ones, sharing your feelings and challenges and always remember that using harmful substances may offer temporary relief but can worsen your blood sugar control and overall wellbeing in the long run.

Limit stimulants: Reduce the intake of caffeine and other stimulants, especially in the evening

Navigating stress involves mindful choices throughout the day. One simple step? Reconsider your caffeine habits. Start by swapping out that afternoon coffee for a herbal tea or warm water with lemon. If you are keen on energy drinks or cola, explore caffeine-free alternatives in the short term, but in the long-term aim to reduce these down or cut them out altogether. Remember, it is not just about better sleep, but also about feeling more balanced during your waking hours. Give your body a chance to unwind and lower stress levels by reducing stimulants, especially in the evening, which will improve your sleep.

>> ACTION POINTS - PRIORITY 2 <<

Limit screen time: The blue light emitted from phones, tablets and computers can interfere with sleep quality

To enhance your sleep quality, it is wise to give your eyes a break from screens before bedtime. The blue light from electronic devices can indeed play havoc with your sleep hormone, melatonin. Instead of watching TV or using your phone before bed, consider reading a book, listening to calming music, or doing gentle stretches. At the very least, if you must be on your phone or tablet prior to sleeping, be sure to turn on the blue light (sometimes called the 'eye comfort') filter. By embracing an evening digital detox, you will move into a more restful state prior to going to bed.

Stay active: Regular physical activity can help regulate sleep patterns

Try to incorporate gentle exercises into your daily routine, maybe a brisk walk or some light stretching in the late afternoon. These activities can naturally boost your mood and tire your body in preparation for rest. Try to avoid high-intensity exercises like sprinting or heavy lifting just before you go to sleep, as they can leave you feeling more wired and less tired.

Limit naps: If you nap during the day, try to keep it short (20-30 minutes) and avoid napping late in the afternoon
While a quick nap can refresh the mind, prolonged or late-afternoon naps might interfere with nighttime sleep. To enjoy the benefits of napping without the drawbacks, set an alarm to limit your naps to 30 minutes. This provides just enough rest to rejuvenate without entering deep sleep cycles. Ideally steer clear of the late afternoon to ensure it does not disrupt your evening sleep rhythm.

Manage stress: Techniques such as deep breathing, meditation, or even gentle yoga before bed can help calm the mind
Managing that stress is key to a restful night, so before turning in, dedicate a few minutes to relaxation. Start with deep, purposeful breaths, inhaling calm, and exhaling worries. The 4-7-8 breathing method can help you drift off to sleep and could be worth trying (I cover this in the section entitled 'Deep Breathing'). If meditation feels right, sit comfortably, and focus on your breathing, letting distractions drift away. Alternatively, gentle yoga poses can help to ease tension.

Stress Relieving Techniques

We have learnt that being truly healthy means taking care of your mental and emotional well-being in addition to your physical health. This approach ensures that you are empowered not only with a body that functions optimally, but also a mind that supports and uplifts.

One aspect that frequently goes unaddressed in type 2 diabetes prevention and reversal is the role of stress. The significance of stress management cannot be overstated, as stress affects your health in many ways over and above playing havoc with your blood sugar levels.

If you are struggling with stress, the following three relaxation methods - journaling, deep breathing and mindfulness - may well help you.

Journaling

In its simplest form, journaling involves writing downs and recording your thoughts, feelings, and experiences. These offer you a personal space to reflect, plan, and communicate with yourself. While it might sound basic, the act of transferring thoughts from your mind to paper can be therapeutic, transformative and, in many cases, quite revealing.

Writing your thoughts down can help you organise them, make sense of experiences, and construct coherent narratives. This process can be helpful in recognising patterns and triggers related to your eating habits or blood sugar level fluctuations. Expressing your emotions in your journal, particularly those that you may have bottled up and kept to yourself, can act as a relief valve that can help you reduce your stress and anxiety levels.

Types of journaling for enhanced wellbeing

- The Gratitude Journal involves noting down things you are thankful for. It can aid you in perspective-shifting, making overcoming challenges feel more surmountable.
- The Food and Blood Sugar Journal is helpful for those that monitor their blood sugar levels. It monitors meals, snacks, medication, physical activity, and blood sugar readings. It can detect relationships between diet, activity, and glucose levels.

- The Reflective Journal is a useful space for deeper introspection. In it, you can explore your feelings, experiences, reactions, and thoughts.
- The Goal-Setting Journal focuses on your future aspirations. It can guide your dietary, physical, and emotional goals.

If you are new to journaling, it can feel daunting - however, it gets easier with practice. You may prefer the tangibility of a physical notebook or perhaps a digital diary or app. There is no need to write essays - as bullet points, lists, or even drawings can convey your thoughts and emotions.

Try to aim for regular entries - daily, every other day or weekly. Find a rhythm that suits you and remember that your journal is your safe space, and it is for you and you alone. Use it to write freely, knowing there is no right or wrong. Going through old entries can show you how much you have grown and what challenges you've overcome.

>> ACTION POINTS - PRIORITY 1 <<

Begin today: Grab a notebook or download a journaling app
Whether you are using a traditional notebook or a digital app, start by writing about your day's feelings or a standout moment. There is no need for detailed narratives, as just a few sentences capturing your emotions or observations will do. Over time, this habit will develop, helping you identify patterns and offering a space for reflection.

Remember, the essence of journaling is authenticity, so write freely without overthinking or judging your words. It is your personal space to explore and understand yourself better.

Commit to consistency: Mark a time in your day, perhaps before bed or during a morning cup of tea, as your journaling moment
To make journaling more effective, create a routine. Choose a specific time each day, like when you have your morning tea or 10 minutes before going to bed. This anchored time will act as a gentle reminder and soon, writing will become a natural part of your day. Your journal is a sacred space; by committing even just a few minutes daily, you will cultivate a therapeutic habit, enabling you to reflect and process your thoughts and emotions more deeply.

>> ACTION POINTS - PRIORITY 2 <<

Stay curious: If you are noting down food and blood sugar readings, remain observant
Every time you record your meals alongside your blood sugar readings, see it as piecing together a personal puzzle. As days turn into weeks, take moments to review your entries. Look for any recurring themes or fluctuations. Perhaps certain foods consistently affect your sugar levels? Paying attention to these details helps you understand your body and make informed choices for your wellbeing.

Reflect and grow: Every few weeks, revisit past entries

Set aside a quiet moment every few weeks to look back over your journal entries. As you read, cherish the positive strides you have made and the patterns of growth and take pride in your journey. Highlight any consistent challenges or areas you feel could be improved. This is not about being hard on yourself, but about understanding where you can further nurture your wellbeing. Think of this reflection as a gentle check-in, a moment to reset, realign and continue your path to a healthier, more balanced you.

Deep Breathing

Deep breathing is about ensuring your oxygen intake is maximised and carbon dioxide is efficiently eliminated. While this might seem simplistic, the depth and rhythm of your breathing can influence various physiological and psychological processes.

Physiologically, deep breathing exercises improve oxygen circulation around the body, which helps cells to receive the oxygen they require to function properly. It can also help in maintaining balanced blood pressure levels as well as improving the digestive process too, ensuring nutrients are effectively absorbed and waste is eliminated properly.

Psychologically, deep breathing can decrease the production and release of stress-related hormones. Deep breathing not only provides extra oxygen to the brain, but also improves emotional regulation and resilience.

While the concept of deep breathing is straightforward to maximise its benefit, ensuring its effective practice requires a little understanding and consistency.

- Diaphragmatic breathing involves breathing deeply by engaging the diaphragm, causing the abdomen to rise and fall instead of the chest, which improves oxygen exchange.

- Counted breathing engages fully with your breath. An example of this is the 4-7-8 technique, which involves inhaling for four seconds through the nose, holding for seven seconds and then exhaling through the mouth for eight seconds. This rhythmic approach helps to create a meditative state, which can help you relax. While deep breathing can be practiced anywhere, your posture can influence its effectiveness and so whether seated or lying down, ensure your spine is straight, allowing unrestricted airflow.

There are several ways that you can make deep breathing a regular and consistent part of your day. In the morning, begin your day with a few minutes of focused breathing, setting a calm and centred tone for the day ahead. Around midday, utilise breathing exercises to refresh part way through the day. In the evening, before retiring to bed, a deep breathing routine can aid relaxation, leading to restorative sleep.

How to practise deep breathing

First, find a quiet, comfortable place to sit or lie down, then close your eyes and take a moment to relax. Inhale slowly through your nose, allowing your abdomen to expand as your lungs fill with air and then exhale gently through your mouth, releasing the air steadily and feeling your abdomen contract. Repeat this cycle for a few minutes, focusing on the rhythm and depth of your breath.

>> ACTION POINTS - PRIORITY 1 <<

Practice awareness: Throughout the day, take moments to become conscious of your breathing
Set gentle reminders on your phone and, when prompted, pause and observe your breath. Feel the rise and fall of your chest or the air passing through your nostrils. Identifying moments when your breathing is shallow can be a sign of tension, so use these moments to take a few deep, calming breaths, helping you to reset.

Set aside dedicated time: Dedicate specific times in your day for focused deep breathing exercises
Start by pinpointing a few moments in your day, perhaps after waking up, during a lunch break, or before bedtime and use these times to sit comfortably, close your eyes and consciously take deep breaths - drawing air deeply into your lungs and exhaling fully.

>> ACTION POINTS - PRIORITY 2 <<

Stay consistent: Aim for daily practice
Just like building a healthy diet, consistency is key with deep breathing exercises so start by setting aside a few minutes each day, perhaps after waking or before sleeping, for focused breathing. As you form this habit, it'll become a natural part of your daily routine.

Utilise technology: Consider apps or online platforms that guide deep breathing exercises

Explore your app store and search for deep breathing or relaxation apps. Many offer guided sessions, visual cues and timers to help you maintain a steady breathing rhythm.

Mindfulness

Mindfulness is the practice of being fully present in the moment. Mindfulness is being aware of your thoughts, emotions, body, and surroundings without judgment.

Practicing mindfulness can have several benefits like reducing cortisol, improving digestion, boosting the immune system, stabilising blood sugar, and lowering blood pressure. It can increase your awareness of thoughts and emotions, resulting in improved concentration and emotional processing.

There are many mindfulness techniques around and no doubt you will find one that suits you perfectly. Here are a few basic techniques to get you started:

- Similar to deep breathing, as mentioned in the previous section, mindful breathing adds an extra layer of awareness. Focus on the sensation of the breath entering and leaving the nostrils, or the rise and fall of the chest or abdomen.
- Body scanning involves mentally scanning your body from top to toe, noting any sensations, any tensions, or any feelings.
- Already covered in a previous section, mindful eating is about truly experiencing your food: its texture, taste, aroma and the sensations of eating. This practice can help you to recognise fullness cues and appreciate smaller portions.

- Mindful walking involves taking a walk, but to let it be free from the usual distractions. Focus on the sensation of each step, the feel of the ground beneath and the rhythm of your stride. Enjoy nature, enjoy being alive.

The great thing about achieving a state of mindfulness is that it does not need to take up much time every day, and can be practiced almost anywhere. So, start small, begin with a few minutes daily, gradually increasing as you grow more comfortable. Aim to include mindfulness in your daily routines. Use a few moments each day for mindful breathing or meditation.

>> ACTION POINTS - PRIORITY 1 <<

Mindful eating challenge: For a week, try eating one meal a day mindfully

Choose one meal each day, perhaps your lunch or dinner, and commit to eating it with no distractions - no TV, no phone, just you and your food. Savour each bite, noticing the textures and flavours. By staying focused on your meal, you can enjoy it more, digest it better, and feel more satisfied, avoiding overeating. After a week, reflect on how this small change has affected your relationship with food and overall wellbeing.

Commit to the practice: Dedicate a few minutes daily for mindfulness

Begin your mindfulness practice by finding a quiet spot, setting a timer for five minutes, and directing your attention to your breath, sensations, and the sounds around you. Try doing this every day at the same time – perhaps in the morning or before bed – creating a routine. Over time, you might extend the duration, but always remember it is the regular practice that matters most.

>> ACTION POINTS - PRIORITY 2 <<

Explore guided sessions: There are many apps and online resources offering guided mindfulness and meditation sessions

There is a selection of websites and apps that offer a range of sessions tailored to different needs, from stress relief to sleep enhancement. Pick one that suits you.

Reflect and journal: After each mindfulness session, spend a minute or two jotting down your experiences, thoughts, or feelings

Keep a notebook handy and simply write down any standout sensations, thoughts, or emotions after each session. Do not aim for perfection; simple, brief reflections are best. Over time, you will notice patterns, growth, and areas that might need attention. By practicing mindfulness, you can deepen self-awareness and keep track of your progress, which motivates you to stay committed.

Step 3 Summary

We are nearly on the home stretch! Thank you for staying with me so far.

I am sure that by reading through step three, you have added to the knowledge gained from steps one and two, and you now have a better understanding of just how 'holistic' your health really is. Diet and exercise alone are not the only areas worthy of consideration when looking to prevent or reverse type 2 diabetes.

Don't forget! You can book a free 15-minute Zoom or phone session with me at **www.diabetessolutions.co.uk/support-sessions** for extra help or to discuss your progress.

As we reach the fourth and final step, I will help you merge all the knowledge from the first three steps into long-lasting habits.

Step 4: Developing Sustainable Habits

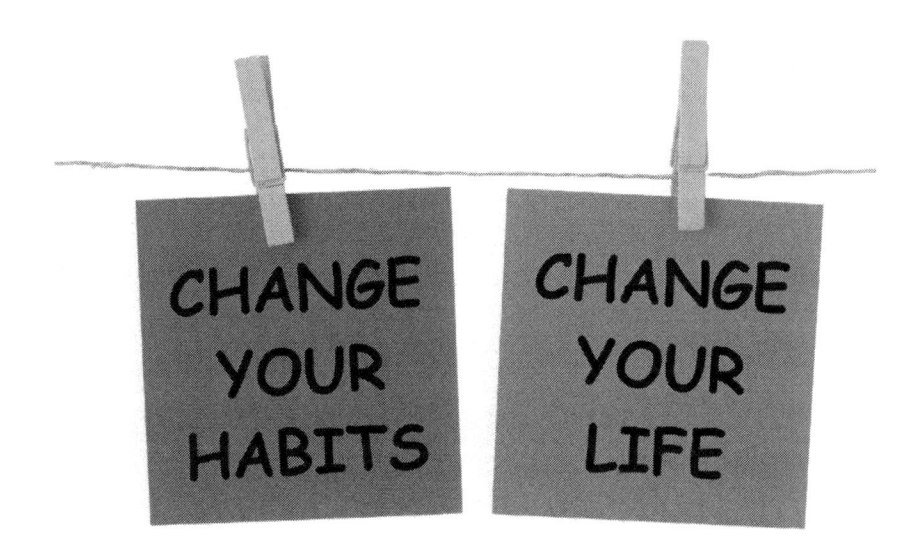

Introduction

Consistency is often seen as the unglamorous part of transformation and, while quick fixes and drastic diet plans might bring temporary success, in my many years of experience (both personally and professionally) they rarely work in the long term. It is only the steady, unyielding power of habit that genuinely brings long-term, positive change.

Understanding the complexity of your actions - why you do what you do - especially when it comes to your health, is crucial. A considerable portion of your daily behaviours are not the result of deep thought or significant conscious decisions, but the culmination of habits that have been formed over many years. In the context of blood sugar control, it is important to understand and be able to harness the power that new and better habits can bring to you.

Why the essence of habit is integral
At a fundamental level, habits are repeated behaviours that have become automatic over time. Consider them as energy-saving shortcuts our brain has developed. They come in handy for tasks like driving, cooking, or tying shoelaces. However, habits can be detrimental when they lead us down a path of poor food choices or sedentary lifestyles.

Together, we need to find ways to convert all the 'Action Points' you have listed down on your worksheets so far into positive daily activities, and new and better habits - only then will they integrate seamlessly into your daily life, without you even consciously thinking about them.

So let us turn the pages and take a closer look at how habits are created, and how you can make habit forming an enjoyable and beneficial experience - in the short, the medium and the long term.

How We Form Habits

Understanding how habits are formed is key in helping you to replace the habits that are proving to be detrimental to your health, with better ones - and this is known as the 'habit loop'.

Here is how the habit loop works:
- **The cue:** This can be the specific time, location, event, emotional state or situation that starts the loop and sparks off an automatic sequence of actions (for example, feeling stressed might be a cue for you to reach for a chocolate bar).
- **The routine:** This is the action or sequence of actions that follows the cue (consuming the chocolate bar would be the routine).
- **The reward:** This is the positive reinforcement received after the routine, which strengthens the habit loop (the momentary pleasure or relief experienced after consuming the chocolate bar serves as the reward).

The brain is incredibly efficient, and to conserve energy, it constantly seeks ways to automate processes. By repeating an action in response to a cue to receive a reward, your brain associates all three components, gradually automating the action until it becomes what we know as a 'habit'.

Every habit follows this same loop so, armed with that knowledge, to improve the habit we then need to recognise the first stage (the cue), replace the second stage (the routine) with a healthier alternative and then enjoy a more sustained and health-benefiting third stage (the reward).

In this example, you would begin by identifying those times when you are feeling stressed and might desire chocolate. You might then choose to replace the chocolate bar with a handful of nuts or a piece of fruit. You have identified the cue, replaced the routine and so will now benefit from a healthier reward.

Here is another example: After every evening meal for many years, you have had a big bowl of ice-cream or a piece of chocolate gateau and you really want to break that habit. It might initially feel challenging to overcome that seemingly deep-seated habit of indulging in desserts after meals. You can change this habit without feeling deprived by gradually incorporating fruit or reducing the amount of ice-cream or cake and pairing it with healthier alternatives.

It is natural to face setbacks while trying to change habits. It is crucial to remember that forming habits is a journey, so occasional indulgences or missed routines shouldn't be seen as major setbacks. Every setback you face offers an opportunity to learn from the experience, to reflect, and then to grow and become stronger.

It sounds simple, but of course we know that in practice, breaking old patterns and establishing new ones can be a challenge. Old habits, especially those formed over years or decades, are often deeply ingrained, but with determination they can be replaced. These new routines, if applied consistently, can benefit your health and help you reshape your habits.

In the free bonus pack, I have put together a 'Habit Loop' worksheet. It will help you identify and consciously adjust any habits that you feel need to be changed.

You can find it at **www.diabetessolutions.co.uk/tkp-bonuspack**

>> ACTION POINTS - PRIORITY 1 <<

Identify your habit loops: List down habits you wish to change and identify the cue, routine, and reward for each

To start, write down the habit you wish to alter. Next, reflect on the cue that prompts this habit - such as a specific time, situation, or emotional state. Next, detail the routine - the actual behaviour you carry out in response to the cue - and finally, the reward you get from it (the feeling or a result). By breaking down this 'habit loop', you gain a clearer insight into why you do what you do and this will start you on the journey towards changing the habit.

Replace, do not erase: Instead of trying to remove an old habit, focus on replacing the routine with a healthier alternative

Changing habits and creating lasting change are often about evolution, not elimination. So, if you have a habit you would like to shift, instead of trying to stop it outright, find a healthier behaviour to take its place. By replacing rather than erasing, you are acknowledging the cue and the reward, but are then adjusting the routine.

Stay consistent: Remember that consistency is important - it is not about being perfect, but about persistent practice

Building new habits is not about getting it right every time, but about being consistent. To put consistency into practice, pick a specific time or trigger for your new behaviour. If you revert to the old routine, then recognise it, acknowledge it, and try to understand why it happened - do not get down or disheartened or feel you have failed. Remind yourself that every day is a fresh opportunity to practise and reinforce your desired new habits.

>> ACTION POINT - PRIORITY 2 <<

Reflect regularly: Each week, assess your progress, recognising both achievements and areas to work on

Choose a moment to review your habit journey so far and write down has gone well. Celebrate those wins and note areas that could use an improvement. This is not about being critical or hard on yourself, but understanding where you are and then refining your approach.

Establishing Positive Habits

We learnt in the previous section about how habits are formed, and it is likely that you are recognising habits in your day-to-day life that you need to address.

The journey to better health and blood sugar control can feel overwhelming because of the number of changes needed. It is okay to feel that way, but with a strategic approach and gradual changes, you can make the process successful and enjoyable.

In the past, you may have tried to make large-scale changes and found out that, while they may have been effective in the short term, they were hard to maintain. Large-scale changes need a lot of energy, motivation, and breaking free from your usual routines to keep going.

Because of this, we are going to look at how small and incremental changes can be integrated into your life with minimal disruption, which should make them more sustainable.

Imagine rolling a small snowball down a snowy hill and as it moves, it gathers more snow, growing in size and momentum. This analogy illustrates the big effect that minor changes can have on your health and life. A single positive habit can set off a chain reaction of improvements, leading to significant long-term benefits.

A small positive change (like reducing the number of teaspoons of sugar in cups of tea or coffee) can then lead to other changes (like choosing water over sugary drinks or a piece of fruit over a chocolate bar), which can then further extend to going out for a 15 minute daily walk. Changes tend to have the proverbial 'snowball effect'.

Unless you can successfully handle (and sustain!) them, I would caution against beginning with making major changes. While perhaps necessary sometimes, making big changes early-on can lead to premature physical or mental exhaustion. For example - suddenly transitioning from a sedentary lifestyle to intense daily workouts can be taxing (possibly leading to injuries or loss of motivation) and therefore, by instead starting with a short daily walk or by gradually reducing sugar intake, you pave the way for a smoother, less stressful transition towards healthier habits.

On the subject of making small and sustainable changes, here are some examples that might resonate with you:

- Before overhauling your entire meal plan, start by making small swaps in your diet.
- Consistently reduce added sugar in your drinks by 10% per week.
- Choose steel-cut oats over refined cereals.
- Gradually increase your intake of vegetables in meals.
- Instead of jumping into a rigorous exercise routine, introduce activity progressively.
- Begin with a 10-minute daily walk, gradually increasing the duration.
- Choose the stairs over the lift when practical.
- Incorporate stretches or basic yoga poses into your morning routine.
- Set weekly or fortnightly check-ins to assess progress.
- Note down how dietary or activity changes make you feel physically and emotionally.
- Reward yourself for consistency, perhaps with non-food treats like a book, a walk in the park, or a relaxing bath.

As you make minor changes, remember that not every adjustment will suit your lifestyle or preferences and so it is essential to be adaptable and recognise when you need to tweak things a little. The goal is to establish habits you can comfortably maintain in the long run, ideally for the rest of your life.

>> ACTION POINTS - PRIORITY 1 <<

Reflect on one small change: Identify one minor dietary or activity change you can integrate this week

This week, try making progress by exchanging a sugary drink for water or taking a short 10-minute walk after dinner. The idea is to choose something that is easily achievable, but that also fits seamlessly into your routine. By focusing on one little change and sticking to it, you will build confidence and pave the way for further positive shifts in your lifestyle and diet. Remember - it is the consistent, small steps that eventually lead to significant changes.

Monitor your feelings: After making the change, note how it affects your energy levels and mood

When you start a new habit, find a quiet moment every day to check in with yourself. Ask questions like, "How do I feel after eating a healthier meal?" or "What is my energy like after going for a walk?" Write down your reflections in a diary or on your phone. It's a great way to connect with the benefits you're experiencing. These observations can become a motivating record of how even small changes can positively impact your wellbeing.

Celebrate: Acknowledge every step, however small, and reward yourself for consistency

Every step forward deserves recognition, so set up a simple tracking system - perhaps a calendar or a journal, to mark your consistent efforts. Reward yourself with something special for reaching milestones like a week of healthy eating or a month of regular exercise. It could be a new book, clothing, a nature walk, or simply some quiet time. These rewards are not just for motivation; they are a reminder of the positive changes you are embedding in your life.

>> ACTION POINT - PRIORITY 2 <<

Stay adaptable: If a change does not resonate, be open to exploring other alternatives

Change is personal, and what works for someone else might not work for you. If you find a new habit is not clicking, do not get disheartened but instead, take a step back and assess why it might not be fitting. Is it too challenging? Why is it not enjoyable? Once you pinpoint the reason, look for an alternative that feels right. Remember, the goal is sustainable positive change, so it is essential to find habits that resonate with you and your unique journey.

Prioritising Consistency

When you are trying to change habits, progress beats perfection every time.

And the key to your progress? Consistency!

Consistency is not about being perfect - it is about commitment to making changes, despite the occasional setbacks. It means staying committed to the practices that improve your health, even when faced with challenges.

You might have heard of "the compound effect". The more you practise healthy habits, the more your wellbeing will improve, similar to how compound interest grows money. Regular, modest, and consistent changes to your habits can result in profound improvements in your health.

Let us not forget the body > mind connection either, as consistent efforts can significantly benefit your mental and emotional wellbeing too - as meeting your daily health goals, however small, can improve your self-esteem and can impart a sense of achievement boosting your confidence.

>> ACTION POINTS - PRIORITY 1 <<

Outline specific goals: Identify specific, achievable health goals for the upcoming week

Start by writing down one or two health goals for the coming week, like taking evening walks or including more vegetables in your meals. Ensure these are manageable within your routine and not overly ambitious. Each evening, review your progress and tweak if necessary. By having a clear vision of your week, you will find it easier to stay on track and see the benefits of consistent, positive habits.

Draft a daily routine: Structure your day to incorporate diabetes-friendly practices

Start with penning down key activities of your day. Next, weave in some good habits (such as having a healthy and balanced lunch or scheduling short breaks to stretch or to walk). Familiarise yourself with this routine and adjust as life happens. With a structured day, following through consistently with practices that support your journey will become easier for you.

>> ACTION POINT - PRIORITY 2 <<

Embrace technology: Explore apps or tools that can help maintain consistency

Begin by browsing your smartphone's app store for top-rated health and type 2 diabetes management tools. Choose one that aligns with your goals, perhaps offering reminders or tracking features. With the right app, you can easily keep up with your healthy habits, like having a personal guide with you all the time.

Habit Linking

Creating better habits is not always about starting from scratch - in fact, sometimes the best approach can be to build on the habits you already have. Leveraging your existing routines can provide a ready-made foundation upon which new, beneficial habits can be constructed.

This is known as 'habit linking'.

The idea behind habit linking is to attach a new practice to a habit you already have. By doing this, new habits can easily slide into your normal routine, which increases their chance of sticking. The key to effective habit linking lies in selecting existing habits that naturally progress into the new ones or share a thematic relevance.

Allow me to explain: Say, for example, you already have the practice of a morning walk, it might be appropriate to link a post-walk glucose check or a balanced breakfast soon after the walk - making the transition between the established habit and the new one feel seamless.

The idea behind linking habits is to use triggers from one habit to remind or prepare you for the next. This connection between actions makes the new habit feel like a continuation, rather than a separate task. While the idea is simple, ensuring success with habit linking requires thought and consistency.

Here are some ways to ensure your linked habits stick:
- Be intentional: it is crucial that the habits you are trying to link are chosen with purpose. The connection should feel logical and seamless to you.
- Start with one pair: While it might be tempting to start linking multiple habits at once, begin with just one pair. Once this pairing becomes second nature, introduce another.
- Visual aids: Sometimes, a visual reminder can help reinforce the connection between linked habits. For instance, keeping your glucose monitor next to your toothbrush or keeping a pot of chia seeds next to your kettle can reinforce the links.
- Regular reflection: Spend some time each week reflecting on how well your linked habits are working. If certain pairings are not sticking, reconsider if they are a logical fit or maybe if they require more intentional reinforcement.

Habit linking can reduce the need to remember each individual task and can also boost your confidence and commitment to change.

>> ACTION POINTS - PRIORITY 1 <<

Identify core habits: Reflect on your day and jot down habits that are already well-established

First, identify the habits you already do effortlessly. (perhaps it is your morning cup of tea or taking your medication after breakfast). Then spend a quiet moment in the evening, reflecting on your day, and list down these 'automatic' actions. By understanding and embracing these fundamental habits, you can smoothly merge and connect new, positive behaviours until they become as natural as your current ones.

Choose a habit pair: Select one new habit you would like to introduce and link it to an existing one
Think of something you already do daily, like having your morning cup of tea. Then, for example, decide that every time you boil the kettle, you will also do 10 press-ups. By pairing these actions, your existing habit becomes a gentle nudge, reminding you of the new one. Over time, this duo becomes second nature, making exercise feel more like part of your everyday rhythm rather than an added task. Remember, the simpler the link, the more effective it will be.

Stay patient and adaptable: Understand that not all habit links might work immediately
When weaving new habits into your routine, patience is key. Imagine you are trying a new recipe; sometimes, you might need a few tweaks to get it just right. Similarly, if a linked habit does not click immediately, do not be disheartened. Take a step back, analyse what might be amiss, and adjust accordingly. It is all about finding the right blend that suits your lifestyle and rhythm. Stay positive and persistent!

>> ACTION POINTS - PRIORITY 2 <<

Visual Reminders: Set up visual cues to strengthen the connection between linked habits

Visual cues can be a real game-changer in strengthening linked habits. For instance, if you are aiming to pair a new dietary choice with your regular morning cup of tea, placing a colourful note or a picture on your tea bag container or fridge door can serve as a gentle nudge. These visual prompts reinforce the link between your established habit and the one you are trying to develop. Over time, seeing that note or image will automatically trigger the paired habit, helping it to become an intrinsic part of your routine.

Weekly reflection: Dedicate time each week to evaluate the progress and success of your linked habits

Setting aside a few moments every day can be immensely beneficial. During this time, think about the linked habits you have been working on. Ask yourself, "Did I effortlessly remember the new habit after the established one?" or "Did the visual cues help?" Reflecting on these questions will offer insights into how effectively your habits are linking and where there might be room for tweaks. Remember, this is all part of the journey of developing new and better habits.

Celebrating Small Wins

As we have learnt, every journey of change comprises a series of big and small steps, and these steps combined should lead you towards your end goal(s). Recognising and celebrating the achievement of every one of these steps will not only make you feel good, but also will help to keep you on the track of sustainable progress.

The big wins are the ones that can sometimes be life-changing, but for the purpose of this section, we are going to focus on the small wins. Even though they may seem insignificant, small wins can have a profound impact on your progress.

Celebrating small victories keeps you moving forward and serves as a reminder that progress, no matter how small, is still progress. These small wins also validate the effort you are making, which boosts your belief in your ability to control your blood sugars.

By celebrating every small win, you are also reinforcing the behaviour that led to that win - making it more likely you will repeat the behaviour. Recalling your past accomplishments can serve as a reminder of your true abilities and the strides you've made.

But what exactly constitutes a small win?

It varies from person to person, but it can include things like choosing a salad over a sugary snack or drinking water instead of a can of fizzy drink. Perhaps you walked an extra 10 minutes than usual or tried a new physical activity? These are all small - but important - wins. Noticing stable blood sugar levels after a meal (which indicates you are learning about how what you eat affects your body and therefore starting to make effective dietary choices) is worthy of celebration as well.

Now that you can identify where you might find the small wins, how might you celebrate them?

The first step in celebrating is to acknowledge the win and take a moment to recognise the effort that went in to achieving it. A dedicated journal to record your wins is helpful. It can motivate you and provide evidence of your progress.

Remember that we discussed the compound effect in a previous section? Well, in the same way, while each small win has its own intrinsic value, their collective impact over time is significant. Imagine each small win as a piece of a larger puzzle; each piece is crucial to completing the picture. Now, I hope you see the value of celebrating small wins.

>> ACTION POINTS - PRIORITY 1 <<

Reflect on your day: At the end of each day, take a moment to reflect and identify any small wins

Pinpoint even the smallest of achievements - maybe you chose a healthier snack, or perhaps you walked a bit more. Celebrating your daily triumphs not only recognises your dedication but also motivates you to keep moving forwards. Remember, every positive step, no matter how small, is progress.

Stay committed: Remember, this journey is a marathon, not a sprint

Think of your journey as a long scenic drive rather than a quick dash. Each small win is like a beautiful landmark along the way, enriching your experience. When confronted with challenges, keep in mind the mindful meals, walks, and positive food choices you have made. Finding inspiration in these moments can re-energise your determination, and celebrating small victories together sets you on the path to a healthier self.

>> ACTION POINTS - PRIORITY 2 <<

Create visual reminders: Consider starting a progress board

Put a corkboard on your wall and then, each time you achieve a small win, pin a note to it. Over time, this board becomes a testament to your consistent efforts, and a visual representation of your journey so far. It is a daily reminder of how far you have come and will help you appreciate every step you have taken. On challenging days, a glance at your progress board can rekindle your determination and focus.

Maintain a journal: Start a dedicated journal to jot down these wins, creating a tangible record of your progress

Find a notebook and designate it as your 'Wins Journal'. Each evening, after your reflection, write down the day's victories, however small. Over time, leafing through its pages will offer tangible proof of your consistent efforts and milestones in your journey.

Re-evaluating Traditional Rewards

We live in a society that sees food as a reward for good behaviour or achieving goals. How many times have you seen someone gain a promotion and then celebrate with cake? It could be that a friend that lost a few pounds then indulged in a 'cheat day' and ate half a dozen biscuits. While these practices seem innocuous, such associations between achievement and reward are counterproductive in the long run, especially if you are trying to get to grips with your blood sugar.

For many, these food-based 'treats' can quickly undo their progress, which then can lead to feelings of guilt, can knock them off course and, sometimes, even causing them to abandon their health goals altogether. To ensure your habits are sustainable, you must change how you think about 'celebration' and break the food-reward cycle.

The next time you feel like celebrating one of the many successes that you will experience over the coming days, weeks, months and years, please remember this image…

do not to reward yourself with food…

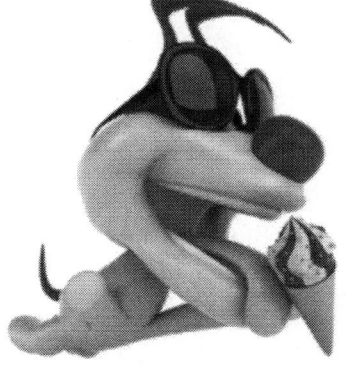

…you are not a dog

Instead of looking at food as a reward for achievement, consider gifting yourself with an experience or a small purchase - perhaps something as simple as an afternoon off to read a book, a day trip to a nearby attraction or maybe a new item of jewellery or clothing. The more you disassociate rewarding yourself with the act of eating, the easier it will become. To celebrate your milestones in your health journey, think about investing in things that support your goals, such as walking shoes or a gym membership.

You might enrol in a course to further develop your knowledge and skills (maybe a nutrition or mindfulness course would be nice, or perhaps even sessions to help you learn a new hobby), or pamper yourself with a spa day, a relaxing bath, or even a meditation session.

These are all positive ways to mark your achievements.

Celebrating differently requires you to experience a mental shift and recognising that rewards do not have to be food-related. By breaking the traditional reward-system norms and habits, you set off a series of positive changes in yourself.

>> ACTION POINTS - PRIORITY 1 <<

Reflect on past celebrations: Think about how you have celebrated achievements in the past

Taking a moment to reflect is enlightening and as you recall past celebrations (perhaps a sweet treat after a weight loss goal or a lavish meal for a fitness milestone) consider how these choices made you feel and their long-term effects. Now, look at alternative rewards that align better with your new and improved health goals. Maybe it is a wellness day, a hobby class, or a health gadget to help you. By comparing your past rewards with healthier options, you can create more thoughtful and beneficial celebrations in the future.

List non-food rewards: Make a list of experiences or items you would consider rewarding

Creating a non-food rewards list can be a game-changer, so grab a notebook or digital note app and brainstorm rewarding experiences or items that you would like (maybe a spa day, a nature hike, or perhaps some new jewellery or clothing). Personalise the list and include rewards for different levels of achievement in your health journey. When you reach milestones, look at the list and select a meaningful reward that recognises your progress.

Regularly update your rewards: As your journey develops, so should your celebrations

As you progress on your health journey, your desires and interests might shift and change. Every few months, take time to revisit your list of rewards and remove any that no longer excites you and add new ones that align with your current aspirations. This ensures your celebrations remain fresh and inspiring. Remember, rewards are personal and should resonate with where you are in your journey, making them meaningful and motivational to help you keep moving forward.

>> ACTION POINT - PRIORITY 2 <<

Share your achievements: Talk about your milestones with friends and family, not only to gain support but also to inspire them
Amplify the importance of your achievements by striking up a conversation with a loved one about them the next time you reach a

milestone. Describe not just the accomplishment itself, but the unique ways you have celebrated. This can then open avenues for encouragement and may even inspire them to think differently about their own milestones. Sharing is not just about your journey; it is a chance to create a ripple effect of a positive change in those around you.

Staying Adaptable

Life is filled with unexpected twists and turns, ups and downs, peaks and troughs. Your ability to adapt to these changes (especially when they affect your health and wellness routines) is important. Instead of quitting, look for alternative methods to continue moving forward and adapt your strategy to the circumstances.

It could be events like holidays, seasonal occasions, family gatherings or even a spontaneous meal that disrupts your routine - and an adaptable mindset will help you enjoy these moments without feeling guilty or overwhelmed. For example, you might go to a party and the only food available is a finger buffet. Rather than worrying unduly and stressing about keeping on track for the coming couple of hours, you can choose to pick the healthiest from the options available, even if what you choose is only the best of the bad choices.

While you may feel it is important to plan your meals, exercises and other routines, ensure your plan has some flexibility. This does not mean straying from your goals but allowing room for adjustments. Understand that it is okay if you do not always stick to the plan. If you have enjoyed a dessert at a family gathering, compensate with a lighter meal or an extra session of physical activity. If you have overindulged at a neighbour's BBQ on Sunday, consider fasting the following day. Instead of being overly strict with yourself, be adaptable and smart.

Instead of perceiving changes as disruptions, consider them as opportunities for growth. This positive mindset makes adapting easier and enjoyable.

Being present in the moment and also recognising changes can help you respond appropriately. Engaging in mindfulness practices such as meditation or deep breathing exercises, that we covered in step three, can help cultivate awareness.

While consistency lays the foundation for habits, adaptability ensures these habits stand the test of time. A wonderful illustration to consider is the humble tree – while it needs to have deep roots (consistency), it should also be able to bend with the wind (adaptability) to avoid breaking. For you, the key is in recognising that consistency should not overshadow adaptability and vice versa. Being overly rigid can lead to stress and burnout, while excessive flexibility might mean drifting away from your objectives. Strive for a harmonious balance where you stay true to your goals, but permit yourself to evolve with changing circumstances.

\>\> ACTION POINTS - PRIORITY 1 <<

Review your routine: Are there areas where you are too rigid or too lax?
Ask yourself: "Are there aspects of my blood sugar control that I consistently overlook, or do I stick too rigidly to one approach, even if it

is not working?" Remember, it is natural for routines to require tweaks over time, but you must listen to your body and learn from experiences. If a part of your routine no longer serves you or feels out of balance, make gentle adjustments. Being adaptable is key to sustainability and effectiveness.

Reframe challenges: Whenever confronted with a change or challenge, practice reframing it positively

However, each challenge also presents an opportunity for growth, so the next time you encounter a setback or unexpected change, pause for a moment. Instead of dwelling on the negatives, ask yourself, "What can I learn from this? How can this experience be a steppingstone for me?" By consciously shifting your perspective, you will cultivate resilience and adaptability.

Anticipating Disruptions

As we learnt in the previous section, life is unpredictable and no matter how well you plan or how disciplined you are, disruptions are inevitable. Unexpected events can temporarily throw you off course, but you can stay on track with the right strategies.

When looking at disruptions, they can be broken down into two different types - predictable and unpredictable.

Events like holidays or scheduled travels are predictable disruptions that you can anticipate and get ready for. Unpredictable disruptions, such as unexpected work commitments or personal events, can catch you off guard. These are often more challenging as they require on-the-spot decision-making and flexibility.

So how can you handle either type of disruption and ensure that you remain on course?

If you know you'll be dining out, try checking the menu beforehand to find foods that match your preferences. Maybe you know that a particular day or week coming up will be busy, or perhaps you are away from your normal environment. In that situation, change your exercise and meal routine beforehand. This could include doing shorter, more intense workouts or preparing and freezing meals ahead of time.

If you are visiting friends or family, perhaps let them know ahead of time what your dietary needs are. Most people are understanding and accommodating and if all else fails, you might carry blood sugar-friendly snacks with you (so even if you face limited food choices, you have something suitable to consume).

When your routine is disrupted for whatever reason, try to maintain your composure and do not stress over the situation. Remember that one-off events do not define your journey; it is the broader picture that matters. Even if it's not perfect, go for the healthiest choice in unexpected scenarios.

If you have consumed something not in your plan, adjust your subsequent meals or add some extra physical activity. Every disruption provides a learning opportunity. Reflect on what happened, understand why it happened, and think about how you can handle it better next time.

While it is important to look at the physical aspect of handling disruptions, it would be remiss of me not to consider the mental and emotional facets too.

From personal experience, I know disruptions can lead to feelings of guilt, disappointment, or discouragement. If you face similar feelings, instead of seeing disruptions as setbacks, view them as part of the journey. One deviation from your routine does not negate all the progress you have made. Avoid thinking that if you have strayed once, the day or week is ruined. It is okay to feel upset or disappointed, but do not dwell on it. Acknowledge your feelings, understand the reasons behind the disruption, and focus on getting back on track.

>> ACTION POINTS - PRIORITY 1 <<

Anticipate disruptions: Look at the week ahead
At the start of each week, take a moment to look at your diary over the 7 days. Spot potential events or situations that might throw you off track, such as social gatherings or work commitments. When you encounter these situations, come up with strategies to navigate them without compromising yourself. This could include preparing a healthy meal ahead of time or scheduling an earlier exercise session. Being one step ahead can make a big difference in fitting your health routine into a busy schedule.

Stay equipped: Always carry a blood sugar-friendly snack and necessary medications with you
Keep healthy snacks (like a handful of nuts or a piece of fruit, alongside any necessary diabetes medications) with you at all times and that way, should an unexpected event extend your day, or a meal gets delayed, you are prepared to maintain stable blood sugar levels.

>> ACTION POINTS - PRIORITY 2 <<

Reflect on past disruptions: Think about a recent disruption
Taking a quiet moment, recall a recent disruption in your blood sugar control routine. Visualise the event, your reaction, and the outcome. Did you respond calmly or with stress? Consider what choices were effective and which were not. Perhaps a meal was missed or an unexpected sweet treat consumed. Being aware of these moments and understanding your reactions helps you build resilience and improve strategies for future disruptions. Embrace these reflections not as criticisms, but as opportunities for learning and growth.

Commit to learning: Every disruption is a learning opportunity
When disruptions occur, view them as lessons and not setbacks. Take a moment to reflect on what happened, asking yourself, "What can I learn from this?" Perhaps it is a change in meal planning, a better way to manage stress, or recognising certain triggers. Transforming disruptions into insights equips you with better strategies for the future and empowers you instead of discouraging you.

Resetting Quickly

While anticipating and preparing for disruptions to your plans is important, it is equally important to understand how to reset quickly when they occur. The speed and effectiveness of your recalibration after disruptions can determine your overall progress. Delayed resets can prolong the negative effects of the disruption.

Consistency is not just about physical actions; it is about mental continuity. A swift reset ensures your motivation and mental commitment remain unbroken. One slight lapse can sometimes lead to a series of deviations from the established routine, so learning to reset quickly helps in avoiding a less-than-ideal situation from worsening.

It is natural to feel disappointment or guilt after a disruption, but dwelling on it can be counterproductive, so recognise the disruption, accept it, focus on the next positive step and keep on moving forwards. You do not always have to return to your full routine immediately, so perhaps begin with a small, manageable action. For instance, if you have deviated from your diet, start your reset with a healthy breakfast, a balanced snack, or a period of intermittent fasting.

It is useful to remind yourself why you started this journey in the first place and look at how far you have come since you started. Take a look at your written goals or any visual aids (like your corkboard) that you might have, as these can reignite your motivation. The most important thing is to give yourself a maximum of 24 hours to recover after noticing a disruption. This allows for a balance between adjusting and not letting the setback last forever.

Be careful of your self-talk, as you are always listening!

Your thoughts influence your actions, so use positive affirmations and remember your past accomplishments. If you have an accountability partner or are part of a support group, let them know about the disruption as they may offer guidance, motivation and practical tips to help you reset.

Having a specific action or series of actions that mark the start of your reset can be useful. This might be a particular exercise, a favourite healthy meal, or even a moment of mindfulness or meditation. Writing down what caused the disruption, how it made you feel, and the actions you took to recover can be a valuable learning tool and source of motivation.

Remember, this journey is not about perfection, but persistence and progress. Recognise that you are only human, and that disruptions are a part of life. Although they can be difficult, disruptions also bring opportunities for growth, learning, and increased resilience. The key lies in your ability to bounce back with determination and a renewed commitment.

>> ACTION POINTS - PRIORITY 1 <<

Avoid self-blame: The next time a disruption occurs, consciously avoid dwelling on guilt

When disruptions arise, it is natural to feel a twinge of guilt. However, dwelling on it will not move you forward. The moment you sense self-blame creeping in, pause and shift your mindset and then remind yourself that everyone faces challenges. Instead of getting stuck in regret, direct your energy towards identifying the next positive step you can take. Whether it is getting back on track with your meal plan or squeezing in a short walk, concentrate on actionable ways to realign with your health goals.

Implement the 24-hour rule: Mark 24 hours after any disruption as a non-negotiable deadline to begin your reset

Using the 24-hour rule can be a game-changer in getting back on track. After any disruption, set a reminder for the same time the next day. Consider this your reminder to take a moment, adapt, and begin anew. Think of it as setting a gentle yet firm deadline for yourself, ensuring that you refocus and continue your path.

Develop a reset ritual: Identify an activity or action that can signify the beginning of your reset process

A reset ritual can be a powerful tool to swiftly bring you back on track. Perhaps it is brewing a cup of herbal tea, taking a five-minute walk, or practicing deep breathing exercises. Find what resonates with you and make it your 'go-to' when you need to refocus. This simple, consistent action signals to your mind that it is time to regroup and start anew and then, over time, the ritual itself will instil a sense of calm and readiness, ensuring you are mentally poised to embrace challenges and continue your journey towards better health.

>> ACTION POINT - PRIORITY 2 <<

Keep your goals to hand: If you haven't already, write down your goals and place them where you can see them daily

Having clear SMART goals can be the anchor to guide you through disruptions. They can help you stay motivated and act as a quick reference point - helping you refocus and reset swiftly whenever you feel off track.

The Power of Positive Reinforcement

Acknowledging your positive choices and the progress you make is important, as acknowledgement plays a big role in our brain's neurological reward system - and that gives us the motivation and drive to keep moving forward.

Our brains have a 'reward system' with pathways that generate pleasure and reward, all to help us survive. When we are rewarded for a behaviour we desire, it increases the chances of repeating that behaviour in the future. Dopamine plays a role in this process.

We covered dopamine (the 'feel-good' hormone) in the section about 'the sugar addiction cycle' - and in the context of sugar addiction, it does indeed work against us - keeping us hooked on sugar. However, as dopamine sits at the heart of the reward system (and its release is associated with pleasure and motivation) we can make it work for us too.

Every positive choice you make and every achievement on your type 2 diabetes journey contributes to your larger goal of being free of the disease or not developing it in the first place. Celebrating choices and accomplishments can activate dopamine, promoting a desire to keep making positive decisions.

In its simplest term - a positive action leads to a positive feeling (courtesy of dopamine), which motivates further positive actions. It is a valuable reinforcing loop.

The more you acknowledge and celebrate achievements, the more dopamine is released and the stronger your motivation becomes to keep striving for your goals. However, you should focus on developing genuine habits that naturally lead to rewarding outcomes, rather than chasing dopamine releases.

Be sure to recognise the positive steps taken on your journey as achievements worth acknowledging. Every time you opt for a balanced meal, decide to take the stairs, or practice mindfulness, you are making headway towards your goal. Being aware of these moments and the dopamine release brings joy and reinforces the significance of these decisions.

\>\> ACTION POINTS - PRIORITY 1 <<

Reflect on achievements: Dedicate time each day to reflect on your positive actions, no matter how small
Celebrating your achievements each day boosts motivation - even small things like making healthier food choices or taking the stairs instead of the lift. Acknowledging any positive steps, no matter how small, will help you gain confidence and stay committed to controlling your blood sugar. It is a simple yet effective way to remind yourself of your progress.

Seek balance: While celebrating achievements is crucial, ensure it does not lead to overindulgence or actions just for the dopamine 'hit'

Seeking balance is all about recognising your successes without going overboard. As you celebrate your achievements, take a moment to reflect on the genuine effort behind them, rather than chasing the next feel-good moment. It is essential to reward yourself in ways that support your health goals, not in ways that will set you back.

>> ACTION POINTS - PRIORITY 2 <<

Journaling: Keep a daily journal to track and celebrate your achievements

Each evening, spend a few minutes jotting down what went well that day – perhaps a new recipe you tried or a walk you enjoyed. As you write, you are not just recording, but also celebrating your daily wins. This act of reflection can become a valuable routine, offering both motivation and a clear view of how far you have come on your health journey. It is a gentle nudge to keep going, even on challenging days.

Mindfulness practices: Engage in mindfulness or meditation to stay connected with your achievements

Begin by setting aside just five minutes a day. Find a quiet spot, close your eyes, take deep breaths, and focus on a recent achievement - visualising the process and the outcome. Feel the joy and pride and immerse yourself in this moment. By recalling the achievement and reinforcing the pleasure it brought, you are enhancing the positive reinforcement. Over time, as this becomes routine, you will find greater satisfaction in your journey, making your commitment even stronger.

Bringing The 4 Steps Together

Congratulations!

You have now navigated the 4 steps of my KISSS Plan. I'm confident you have gained valuable knowledge, have lots of great Action Points to work on, and are now ready to put them into practice.

Your strategies will probably evolve as time passes, so be adaptable and keep the KISSS Plan book at hand to refer back to at any time.

Before we wrap up, let us quickly recap each step.

Step 1: Nutrition

In Step 1, we laid the foundation by acquiring knowledge and understanding the "what" and the "why" of type 2 diabetes prevention and reversal. You learnt about the fundamentals of nutrition, the impact of sugar on blood sugar levels, and the importance of balanced eating. You can now make more informed and healthier food decisions by understanding the difference between natural and added sugars. You also discovered how to interpret food labels, identify hidden sugars, and understand the role of sugar alternatives.

In each section of step 1, we looked at ways to apply what was learnt into your daily life. The 'Action Points' at the end of each section are for you to choose, personalise and work on according to your current needs and ability. Keep your worksheets where you can easily refer to them. Put your Action Points into practice. Be sure to review them regularly and adjust/update them as needed.

Step 2: Get Moving!

In Step 2, we explored the importance of physical activity in achieving better health. You learnt that to prevent and reverse type 2 diabetes, it is important to have a balanced approach to health that includes nutrition and physical activity. You learnt practical tips to incorporate movement into your daily life and you created several Action Points that should help you make regular movement and/or exercise a sustainable part of your routine.

Step 3: Holistic Wellbeing

Step 3 emphasised that true health is holistic. It encompasses your physical, mental, and emotional wellbeing - and requires addressing all aspects of your life, not just diet and exercise. Balancing and maintaining a healthy life involves managing stress, getting enough sleep, and being emotionally resilient. We explored ways to improve overall wellbeing through mental and emotional health.

Step 4: Creating Sustainable Habits for Life

In the final step, we discussed the importance of building habits that last a lifetime. We looked at practical strategies to help you create new, better, and sustainable habits. You learnt that health is a lifelong journey, and quick fixes rarely lead to lasting results. Sustainable habits are the key to long-term health, and we looked at how these are the building blocks of sustainable health improvement - and by adopting healthier habits, you will make positive changes to your diet and lifestyle, achieving your goal of preventing or reversing type 2 diabetes.

Bonus Pack

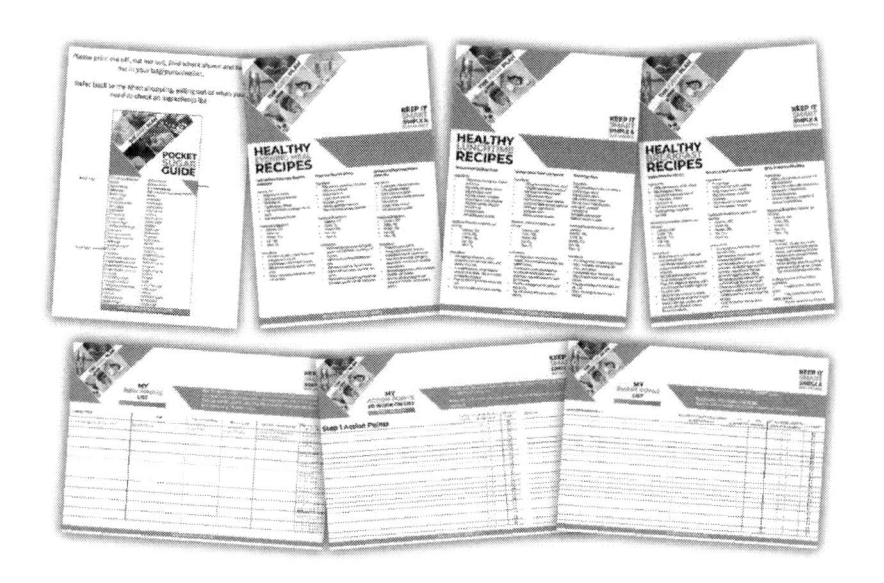

- Over 100 free healthy breakfast, lunch and evening meal recipes
- Free SMART goals worksheet
- Free 'Action Points' worksheet.
- Free Habit-Forming worksheet.
- Free sugar names pocket guide

To access your free bonus content, simply visit the following link: www.diabetessolutions.co.uk/tkp-bonuspack

Free 15 Minute Consultation

Would a free 15 minute chat help you?

I set aside time each week to offer free 15-minute Zoom or phone consultations to help those who have questions or concerns regarding their diet, nutrition, preventing type 2 diabetes, or reversing pre-diabetes and type 2 diabetes.

If that interests you and you feel it would be of benefit, then it would be great to have a friendly, informal, and no-obligation chat.

You can book a free 15 minute Zoom or phone session with me at: www.diabetessolutions.co.uk/support-sessions

If you would like a longer session and would like to book a 30 minute, 60 minute or 90 minute Zoom consultation with me, you can find those options there too.

Regular 121 Help

Would you like me to help you on a regular 1-2-1 basis?

Via Zoom, I work with clients globally, providing support and education in preventing or reversing pre-diabetes and type 2 diabetes.

If you feel I could help you too on a 121 basis, then let's have a chat.

Please contact me at: www.diabetessolutions.co.uk/contact

Free Online Reversal Assessment

Take my free online assessment and find out in just three minutes if you might be able to reverse your Type 2 Diabetes.

I have put together a free type 2 diabetes reversal assessment that should take you no more than three minutes to complete.

Based on your answers to the questions, at the end of the assessment, you will be given a percentage score.

The higher the score, the more likely the chance that you might reverse your type 2 diabetes.

Curious? Then why not take the assessment?

You can find it here: www.t2dra.com

Keep In Touch!

It would be great to keep in contact.

I would like to drop you interesting and relevant information via email from time to time, that may well help you on your type 2 diabetes prevention/reversal journey.

I promise to be respectful of your data, to treat it in accordance with current data protection legislation and to not permit third parties to access it.

To become a Diabetes Solutions subscriber for free, please go to: www.diabetessolutions.co.uk/subscribe

Closing Thoughts

I sincerely hope that my book has both enlightened you and motivated you to want to make changes in your life, wherever you are in relation to type 2 diabetes.

Going from where you are now to where you want to be may not be a straightforward journey, as I have mentioned.

However, the destination of improved health and quality of life that you will experience (together with everything that goes along with that) in the coming weeks, months and years is absolutely worth the effort that you put in right now.

I wish you every success for the future, and will leave you with one last, abiding thought… Strive for progress and not perfection. Every step that you make in the right direction is a step in the right direction - no matter how small.

The journey of a thousand miles begins with the first step.

So, make that first step, **right now.**

Neil

www.diabetessolutions.co.uk

Glossary

A

A1C test: A blood test used to diagnose type 1 and type 2 diabetes and gauge how well diabetes is being managed by measuring average blood sugar level over the past three months.

Acanthosis Nigricans: Dark, velvety patches of skin in the creases and folds of the body.

Adenosine Triphosphate (ATP): A molecule that stores and transfers energy within cells.

Adiponectin: A protein hormone involved in glucose regulation and fatty acid breakdown, often found at lower levels in individuals with obesity-related insulin resistance.

Aerobic exercise: Physical activities that increase heart rate and improve the efficiency of the cardiovascular system.

Alpha-glucosidase inhibitors: Medications that slow the digestion of carbohydrates in the intestines, thus helping to lower blood sugar levels.

Amino acids: organic compounds that combine to form proteins, playing a vital role in constructing and repairing tissues, supporting neurotransmitter functions and participating in various metabolic processes within the body.

Amylin: A hormone produced by the pancreas that regulates the timing of glucose release into the bloodstream post meals and helps control appetite.

Antihyperglycemic: Medications or actions designed to lower elevated blood glucose levels.

Antioxidants: Molecules that help protect the body against free radicals, which can damage cells.

Asthenia: Constant fatigue attributed to insufficient glucose reaching the cells

Autonomic neuropathy: A type of neuropathy affecting the nerves that manage involuntary functions like heart rate, blood pressure and digestion.

Autophagy: the process in which cells break down and recycle damaged components and debris to maintain proper function and health.

B

Balanced diet: A diet comprising the right quantity and proportion of foods from all food groups, ensuring that the body receives all essential nutrients.

Baseline blood sugar: The amount of sugar in the bloodstream upon waking, before any food or physical activity.

Beta cells: Cells located within the pancreas, responsible for producing and releasing insulin.

Blood glucose: Also known as blood sugar, it refers to the concentration of sugar present in the blood. it is the main source of energy for the body's cells.

Blood glucose diary: A record used by individuals with diabetes to track their blood sugar levels, often alongside food intake, exercise and insulin doses.

Blood glucose meter: A device that measures and displays the amount of sugar in a small sample of blood, usually from your fingertip.

Blood sugar spike: A rapid increase in blood glucose levels, which can result from food, stress, or other factors.

Body Mass Index (BMI): A measure used to determine if a person has a healthy body weight for their height.

Bolus insulin: A type of fast-acting insulin administered around meals to counteract the rise in blood sugar that comes with eating.

C

C-Peptide: A molecule created when insulin is produced. Testing C-peptide levels can give insights about a person's insulin production.

Caloric intake: The number of calories consumed through food and drink over a period.

Candidiasis: Yeast infections caused by excessive sugar in the blood and urine.

Carbohydrate counting: A method used to manage blood sugar levels by counting the number of carbohydrates consumed.

Carbohydrates: One of the primary food categories, it includes sugars, starches and fibres. Carbohydrates impact blood glucose levels the most.

Cardiovascular health: Pertaining to the health of the heart and blood vessels.

Cell: The basic structural and functional unit of living organisms.

Cholesterol: A waxy substance found in the blood. People with diabetes are advised to monitor their cholesterol levels due to increased risk of heart disease.

Circadian rhythms: Physical, mental and behavioural changes that follow a daily cycle, influenced by natural light and darkness.

Continuous Glucose Monitor (CGM): A device that tracks blood glucose levels throughout the day and night.

Cortisol: A hormone produced in the body, often in response to stress. Elevated levels can impact weight and blood sugar management.

Cytokines: Small proteins released by cells, playing a key role in cell signalling, especially during immune responses.

D

Dawn phenomenon: An early morning rise in blood sugar levels, which can be a response to the body's natural overnight release of hormones.

Diabetes burnout: A state of mental and physical exhaustion where individuals become tired of managing their diabetes and sometimes ignore their treatment plan.

Diabetic dermopathy: Skin changes, often in the form of light brown, scaly patches, commonly seen in older individuals with a history of diabetes.

Diabetic foot ulcer: An open sore or wound, commonly located on the bottom of the foot, in people with diabetes.

Diabetic myonecrosis: A rare complication of diabetes leading to muscle damage.

Diabetic nephropathy: Kidney damage or disease caused by diabetes, which can lead to kidney failure if not treated.

Diabetic neuropathy: A complication involving nerve damage because of prolonged elevated blood glucose levels, often causing pain or numbness in the hands and feet.

Diabetic retinopathy: Diabetes-related damage to the eyes' blood vessels, which can cause vision issues or blindness if untreated.

Dipeptidyl Peptidase-4 (DPP-4) inhibitors: Oral diabetes medications that help increase insulin production and decrease glucose production.

Diuretic: Medications often prescribed to individuals with diabetes to eliminate excess salt and water from the body. Can also refer to drinks that encourage urination, like coffee.

Dyslipidaemia: An abnormal amount of lipids (cholesterol and/or fats) in the blood, commonly found in people with diabetes.

E

Electrolyte: A mineral in the body that carries an electric charge and is essential for maintaining physiological functions such as muscle contractions and fluid balance.

Emotional eating: The act of consuming food in response to emotional needs rather than physical hunger.

Endocrine system: A collection of glands that produce hormones regulating metabolism, growth, tissue function and mood.

Endorphins: Chemicals produced by the body to relieve stress and pain. They can produce a feeling of euphoria similar to that produced by opioids.

Energy balance: The balance between calories taken in through diet and calories expended through physical activity.

Euglycemia: A state where blood glucose levels are within the accepted and targeted range.

F

Fasting blood sugar: The measure of glucose in the bloodstream after refraining from eating for about 8-10 hours.

Fats: Macronutrients essential for energy and supporting cell growth. They also help protect organs and absorb nutrients.

Fatty acids: Fatty acids are long chains of carbon, hydrogen and oxygen atoms that make up fats and can be used by the body for energy and various cellular functions.

Fatty liver disease: Accumulation of fat in the liver, often linked to insulin resistance.

Foot screening: Regular checks on the feet of those with diabetes to prevent complications, given the risk of ulcers and neuropathy.

Free radicals: Unstable molecules that can damage cells and contribute to ageing and diseases.

G

Gastroparesis: A complication where nerve damage affects the stomach's muscles, slowing or preventing the movement of food through the gastrointestinal tract.

Ghrelin: Often termed the 'hunger hormone', it signals the brain to initiate feelings of hunger.

Gingivitis (or Periodontitis): Gum infections caused by a compromised ability to fight bacteria.

Glomerular Filtration Rate (GFR): A measure of how well the kidneys are filtering wastes and excess substances.

Glucagon: A hormone released by the pancreas when blood sugar is too low, prompting the liver to convert stored glycogen into glucose.

Gluconeogenesis: A pathway that enables glucose to be produced from sources other than carbohydrates (like proteins or fats).

Glucose metabolism: The processes by which the body handles and processes sugar.

Glucose tolerance test: A procedure measuring the body's ability to metabolise sugar by monitoring glucose levels after consuming a sugary solution.

Glycaemic Index (GI): A ranking of carbohydrates in foods according to how they affect blood glucose levels.

Glycerol: the backbone of triglycerides, it binds with three fatty acid molecules to create the tri-structure.

Gratitude journal: A tool used for wellbeing, focusing on recording aspects of life one is thankful for, promoting a positive mindset.

Growth Hormone: A hormone involved in cellular repair, growth and metabolism.

H

HBA1C test: A blood test used to diagnose type 1 and type 2 diabetes and gauge how well diabetes is being managed by measuring average blood sugar level over the past three months.

Holistic wellbeing: An approach that considers the whole person – body, mind, spirit and emotions – in the quest for optimal health and wellness.

Homeostasis: the process by which the body maintains a stable internal environment, despite external changes, to ensure optimal functioning of its systems.

Hyperglycaemia: A condition characterised by an excessively high level of glucose in the blood, commonly seen in individuals with diabetes.

Hyperinsulinemia: A condition characterised by excess insulin levels in the bloodstream

Hyperpigmentation: Patches of darkened skin, indicative of insulin resistance or hormonal imbalance.

Hypoglycaemia: A condition where the level of glucose in the blood drops below normal, often due to excessive insulin or a lack of dietary glucose.

I

Incretin: Hormones that stimulate insulin secretion in response to meals.

Islets of Langerhans: Clusters in the pancreas made up of several cell types, including insulin-producing beta cells.

Insulin: A hormone produced by the pancreas that regulates the amount of glucose in the blood. It allows cells to use glucose for energy.

Insulin peak: The time frame when insulin's glucose-lowering effect is strongest.

Insulin pen: A pen-like device offering a convenient method to inject insulin, with cartridges typically replaceable.

Insulin pump: A wearable device providing continuous insulin delivery through a small catheter, reducing the need for multiple injections.

Insulin resistance: A condition in which the body's cells become resistant to the effects of insulin, leading to increased blood sugar levels.

Insulin sensitivity: How receptive the body is to the effects of insulin. Increased insulin sensitivity reduces the risk of type 2 diabetes.

J

Journaling: The practice of recording thoughts, feelings and experiences in written form for reflection, planning and personal growth.

K

Ketoacidosis: A potentially life-threatening condition characterised by high blood sugar and the presence of ketones in the urine, resulting from insufficient insulin.

Ketones: Compounds produced when the body begins using fat instead of carbohydrates for energy due to low insulin levels.

L

Latent Autoimmune Diabetes in Adults (LADA): A form of diabetes that shares characteristics with both type 1 and type 2 diabetes, often diagnosed in adulthood

Leptin: A hormone that signals the feeling of fullness and suppresses hunger.

M

Macronutrients: Essential nutrients required in significant amounts in our diet. They include carbohydrates, proteins and fats.

Macronutrient ratio: The balance of carbohydrates, proteins and fats in a diet.

Macrovascular: Relating to the larger blood vessels in the body. Macrovascular complications in diabetes include cardiovascular diseases.

Meal planning: Organising meals and snacks ahead of time to ensure balanced nutrition.

Meglitinides: A class of drugs that stimulate the pancreas to release more insulin.

Melatonin: A hormone produced by the pineal gland that regulates sleep-wake cycles.

Metabolic health: Refers to the optimal functioning of the body's metabolic processes, often associated with balanced blood sugar levels and proper insulin function.

Metabolic rate: The rate at which the body expends energy or burns calories.

Metabolic syndrome: A cluster of conditions, including increased blood pressure, high blood sugar and abdominal obesity, that increase the risk of heart disease, stroke and type 2 diabetes.

Metabolism: A set of chemical reactions in the body that transform food into energy required for survival and functioning.

Metformin: A frequently prescribed medication for type 2 diabetes, aiding in lowering blood sugar levels by improving insulin sensitivity.

Microbiome: the community of microorganisms (including bacteria, fungi, viruses, and other microbes) that inhabit the human gut.

Micronutrients: A vital substance required in small amounts by the body for proper growth and good health.

Microvascular: Relating to the smaller blood vessels in the body. Microvascular complications in diabetes include retinopathy, nephropathy and neuropathy.

Mind-body connection: The interrelationship between our thoughts, feelings and bodily functions.

Mindful eating: Paying full attention to the eating process, being aware of colours, smells, textures, and flavours of food.

Mindfulness: A mental practice focusing on being fully present, aware of where we are and what we are doing, without being overly reactive.

Mindfulness practices: Techniques that encourage present-moment awareness, often used for stress reduction.

Minerals: Inorganic substances essential for various physiological functions and are obtained through the diet.

Mitochondria: Small structures within cells responsible for producing energy.

N

Nutrient density: A measure of the nutrients a food provides relative to the calories it provides.

Neurotransmitter: Chemical messengers that transmit signals in the brain and play roles in mood as well as bodily and cognitive function.

O

Oral glucose tolerance test (OGTT): A test in which glucose is given and blood samples are taken afterward to determine how quickly glucose is cleared from the blood.

Omega-3 fatty acids: A type of fat that has been linked to several health benefits, including reducing inflammation and heart disease risk.

Oxidative stress: An imbalance between free radical production and the body's ability to counteract or detoxify their harmful effects through neutralisation by antioxidants.

P

Pancreas: An organ located in the abdomen that plays a crucial role by producing enzymes and hormones like insulin to regulate blood sugar levels.

Peripheral Artery Disease (PAD): A condition where the blood vessels, typically in the legs, become narrowed, reducing blood flow.

Peripheral neuropathy: nerve damage caused by prolonged exposure to high blood sugars, affecting the delicate nerve fibres.

Physical activity: Any movement that makes your muscles work and requires your body to burn calories. it is essential for overall health and is especially important for managing and potentially reversing type 2 diabetes.

Phytosterols: naturally occurring compounds found in plant cell membranes that have health benefits when consumed.

Polydipsia: Excessive thirst and fluid intake, a common symptom of elevated blood sugar levels.

Polyphagia: Increased hunger caused when the body is unable to effectively use glucose as a fuel source.

Polyuria: The need for frequent urination

Portion control: Monitoring the amount of food consumed in one sitting to ensure it aligns with nutritional needs.

Postprandial blood sugar: The amount of glucose in the blood, typically measured about two hours after eating.

Prediabetes: A condition where blood sugar levels are consistently high but not yet within the diabetes range, indicating an increased risk of developing type 2 diabetes.

Protein: A macronutrient essential for building and repairing tissues, making enzymes and supporting many body functions.

Pruritus: Itchy rashes, commonly found in moist areas such as the armpit or groin, caused by bacteria and yeast feeding excessive sugar in the blood and urine.

R

Reactive hypoglycaemia: Low blood sugar occurring within four hours after a meal.

Reflective journal: A form of journaling focused on introspection and reflection on personal experiences and feelings.

Resetting: Realigning oneself to previously set goals and habits after a disruption or break.

Resistant starch: A type of starch that is not fully broken down and absorbed, potentially beneficial for blood sugar control.

Restorative sleep: Sleep that promotes physical and psychological restoration.

S

Satiety: The satisfying feeling of fullness after consuming food, playing a crucial role in regulating food intake.

Saturated fats: Type of fat typically solid at room temperature, found primarily in animal sources.

Somogyi effect: A rebound effect where a significant drop in blood sugar is followed by a rapid rebound high, often caused by excessive insulin doses or missed meals.

Starch: A carbohydrate found in many plants, consisting of numerous glucose units bonded together, primarily serving as an energy storage compound.

Stress: The body's response to any change requiring an adjustment or reaction.

Sugar alcohols: Types of sweet carbohydrates that come from plants and have a chemical structure that partially resembles sugar and alcohol.

Sulfonylurea: A medication category prompting the pancreas to produce more insulin, often prescribed in early stages of type 2 diabetes.

T

T-cells: A type of white blood cell that is essential for immune responses.

Thiazolidinediones (TZDs): Medications that improve insulin sensitivity.

Tissue: A group of cells that perform a similar function.

Trace elements: A chemical element required in minute amounts by living organisms for proper physiological functioning.

Triglycerides: A type of fat often found in the bloodstream. Elevated levels can increase the risk of heart disease.

Type 1 diabetes: An autoimmune condition where the body's immune system attacks insulin-producing beta cells, leading to little or no insulin production.

Type 2 diabetes: A chronic condition where the body either resists the effects of insulin or does not produce enough insulin to maintain a normal glucose level.

U

Unsaturated fats: Healthy fats, usually liquid at room temperature and found in plants.

Urine ketone test: A test that checks for the presence of ketones in the urine, indicating uncontrolled diabetes.

V

Vascular: Pertaining to blood vessels. In diabetes, vascular complications are of significant concern.

Visceral fat: Fat stored in the abdominal area, closely linked to insulin resistance and type 2 diabetes.

Vitamins: organic compounds essential for bodily functions and health, obtained primarily through food.

W

White noise machine: A device that produces consistent ambient sound, used to mask disruptive noises for improved sleep.

Whole foods: Foods that are unprocessed and unrefined, or processed and refined as minimally as possible.

Whole grains: Grains that include the entire grain kernel, i.e., the bran, germ and endosperm.

X

Xerosis: Dry skin caused by dehydration.

Xerostomia: Dry mouth caused by reduced or absent saliva flow, which can be a side effect of high blood sugars.

About The Author

Neil D'Silva is a distinguished nutritionist specialising in the areas of type 2 diabetes prevention and reversal. His journey into nutrition combines personal and professional aspects, shaping his unique perspective. He is also founder of Diabetes Solutions - a wellbeing company dedicated to helping pre-diabetics and type 2 diabetics in their quest for better health.

In his earlier years, Neil navigated the challenges of weight gain and health issues. However, everything changed for Neil in 2012 when his father passed away. This event, along with his own health issues, sparked his passion for health, nutrition, and type 2 diabetes. With an extensive array of qualifications, Neil has established himself as an authority in the field.

As Neil continues to make strides in the field of nutrition, he is also venturing now into authorship with The KISSS Plan - aiming to share his wealth of knowledge to a global audience with the genuine commitment to see an end to type 2 diabetes (and the suffering it causes) across the world.

Find out more at www.diabetessolutions.co.uk

Printed in Great Britain
by Amazon

11198315-8200-4d8a-867a-8dfb40f4a73eR01